Understanding EMG

Understanding EMG

Making sense of nerve conduction and EMG in clinical practice

Andrew Michell
Consultant in Clinical Neurophysiology,
Department of Clinical Neurophysiology,
Addenbrooke's Hospital,
Cambridge, UK

OXFORD
UNIVERSITY PRESS

OXFORD
UNIVERSITY PRESS

Great Clarendon Street, Oxford, OX2 6DP,
United Kingdom

Oxford University Press is a department of the University of Oxford. It furthers the University's objective of excellence in research, scholarship, and education by publishing worldwide. Oxford is a registered trade mark of Oxford University Press in the UK and in certain other countries

First published 2013

British Library Cataloguing in Publication Data
Data available

ISBN 978–0–19–959550–1

Preface

Understanding EMG has been written for clinicians who need to understand when to request nerve conduction studies and EMG, and how to interpret the results in light of the clinical presentation. The focus throughout the text is on clinically useful concepts, which are reinforced and expanded in the case discussion section at the end where roles and shortcomings of electrodiagnosis are considered in common clinical settings.

The book starts with the essentials of neuromuscular anatomy and physiology required for a fundamental understanding of electrodiagnosis. This is genuinely required for clinical interpretation of the tests, not just provided for the enthusiast! The electrodiagnostic examination is then considered along three conceptual axes that define both performance of the examination and its interpretation:

1. Pathology, determined by recognition of familiar patterns of electrodiagnostic findings.
2. Localization of the abnormality.
3. Timing of the examination in relation to evolution of pathology.

Of the three, it is arguably the time course of evolution of electrodiagnostic findings that is most important for referring clinicians to understand.

It is often stated that the electrodiagnostic examination is an extension to the clinical examination. This is true, but it is less widely appreciated that, just like its clinical counterpart, some findings are 'hard' reliable predictors of pathology, whilst others are 'soft' and thus to be given less weight in drawing conclusions. An attempt is made to convey this in order that readers start to develop a better appreciation of how results should be weighted and interpreted. Not everyone will agree with my assessment of 'hard' versus 'soft' findings, but that they exist is undeniable, and my aim in chapter 10 is to provoke considered interpretation of results. There are a number of common situations in which the clinical presentation and electrodiagnostic results may seem to be at odds with one another, and these are considered in this chapter too—if you only have time to read one chapter, it is this one I would recommend.

Electrodiagnosis is of course a consultation, not just a test, since the conclusion represents a judgement about interpretation of findings in light of the clinical presentation and differential diagnosis. Ultimately the physician performing the electrodiagnostic examination is best placed to weigh up its findings, so difficult cases should be discussed whenever possible.

One goal of this book is to provide enough detail to be practically useful, whilst sticking to basic concepts and avoiding superfluous detail or the need for prior expertise. There is no discussion of how to actually perform the tests since this is best done at the bedside if required. The need for extensive knowledge of neuroanatomy has been minimized with the 'Anatomy Buster' (Chapter 13). I have included a fairly extensive explanation of EMG since this is often poorly understood, and is fundamental to understanding the strengths and limitations of the technique and what it all means.

In preparing this book I have of course had help and encouragement. I am particularly grateful for the insightful teaching of many during my training, especially Drs Nick Murray and Shelagh Smith at the National Hospital for Neurology and Neurosurgery, Queen Square, London. Several colleagues have given opinions, encouragement, and comments on various stages of the manuscript including, in particular, Drs Charlotte Brierley and John McHugh, although any mistakes are my own. My publishers, Oxford University Press, have been very patient and helpful, particularly Peter Stevenson, Sarah MacBean, Eloise Moir-Ford, Abigail Stanley, and Nic Williams. Finally, of course my wife, Jo, and young family have been very tolerant of my numerous late nights working in 'level eight', so the book is dedicated to them.

Contents

Section 1

Chapter 1

Essential Anatomy and Physiology

Key points

- Resting membrane potential is determined largely by high permeability to K^+, and is −70mV to −90mV, negative inside.
- If the depolarizing potential reaches threshold it triggers the opening of voltage-gated Na^+ channels, and thus an action potential.
- Most axons in a human nerve are of small diameter (<6μm) and are not measured by routine nerve conduction studies.
- Conduction velocity is fastest in large diameter axons, and in those that are myelinated.
- A presynaptic influx of Ca^{2+} triggers acetylcholine release at the neuromuscular junction, generating a postsynaptic end-plate potential which triggers an action potential if threshold potential is reached.
- The number of muscle fibres in a motor unit is highly variable depending on the muscle and the presence of pathology.
- Electromyography (EMG) is dominated by type I rather than type II muscle fibre activity.
- The force of muscular contraction depends on the number of muscle fibres activated and their firing rate.

Nerve conduction studies and **EMG** can inform us about pathology affecting the anterior horn cell, nerve roots, plexus, peripheral nerve, neuromuscular junction, and finally the muscle. Large-diameter motor and sensory axons are tested. To interpret peripheral neurophysiological studies correctly, and understand the strengths and weaknesses of different examination techniques, it is necessary to have a basic understanding of neuromuscular anatomy and physiology.

Resting Membrane Potential

Excitable membranes are composed of impermeable lipid bilayers that are spanned by protein channels which selectively allow the passage of specific ions. The potential difference between the intracellular and extracellular spaces is termed the membrane potential. It is dictated primarily by the selective permeability of the membrane together with the presence of many negatively charged proteins within the cell. The Na^+/K^+ pump makes only a small contribution to **resting membrane potential**.

Chemical gradients of ions exist across the cell membrane, with high K^+ and low Na^+ concentrations inside the cell, and the reverse in the extracellular space. In the resting state the membrane is highly permeable to K^+ ions, which move across the membrane freely until the chemical gradient driving these ions out of the cell is balanced by the electrical gradient keeping them in, at which point they have reached their equilibrium potential (–75mV for K^+). The membrane potential depends almost entirely on the sum of the equilibrium potentials for K^+, Na^+, and Cl^-, weighted for their permeabilities. In practice, this means that the resting membrane potential is dominated by K^+ because of its high permeability, and is –70mV to –90mV, negative inside.

Action Potentials

At the synapse some neurotransmitters are excitatory, causing an influx of Na^+ and Ca^{2+}, thereby depolarizing the membrane, termed the generator potential. Other neurotransmitters are inhibitory, and resist this **depolarization** by increasing K^+ and Cl^- conductance. The type of channel and neurotransmitter varies, but the principles of excitation remain the same. When the generator potential reaches **threshold** it triggers the opening of voltage-gated Na^+ channels, resulting in further depolarization due to the influx of Na^+. This triggers a cascade of further rapid depolarization whereby any remaining voltage-gated Na^+ channels also open: the depolarizing upstroke of the **action potential** (Fig. 1.1).

Voltage-gated Na^+ channels are time-locked, and close after just 1–2ms. This is accompanied by the reopening of K^+ channels, which eventually leads to a slight **hyperpolarization** of the membrane. Interestingly, in human nerves there are many Na^+ but few K^+ channels at the nodes of Ranvier. The inactivation of Na^+ channels determines the absolute refractory period of that neuron, during which a second stimulus will not trigger an action potential, and this is followed by a relative refractory period. The membrane permeability to Ca^{2+} follows a similar time course to K^+, the resultant transient influx of Ca^{2+} at the **motor nerve** terminus being essential for neuromuscular junction function.

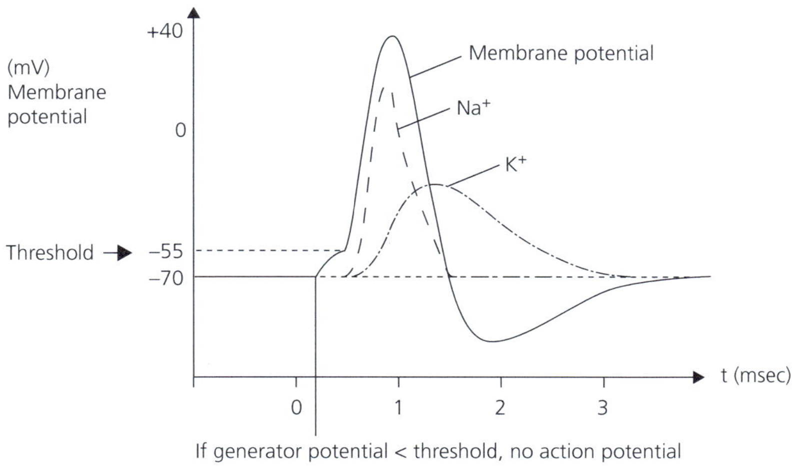

Figure 1.1 The change in Na^+ and K^+ conductance and time course of the nerve action potential.

Adapted from *Electromyography and Neuromuscular Disorders: Clinical-Electrophysiologic Correlations*. Copyright (1998), with permission from Elsevier.

Myelin insulates the nerve, resulting in spread of depolarization much further along the nerve than if it was unmyelinated. Once the next node of Ranvier is depolarized sufficiently to exceed threshold the same cascade occurs, and thus the action potential is propagated. This 'saltatory conduction' allows conduction velocities exceeding 50m/s in large-diameter myelinated fibres, compared to <5m/s in those that are unmyelinated.

With electrical stimulation of a nerve the depolarization beneath the **cathode** exceeds threshold potential, resulting in the opening of voltage-gated Na^+ channels and the propagation of an action potential in both directions along the nerve, away from the cathode.

Nerve Anatomy: Function, Disability, and Prognosis

Numbers and types of axon

Most nerves are made up of many different types and diameters of axon, which may be classified according to their size, degree of myelination, whether they carry sensory or motor information, or whether they are part of the somatic or autonomic nervous systems (Table 1.1).

Human nerve biopsies show there are about 10,000 axons/mm^2 cross-sectional area, thus there are in the region of 100,000 or more fibres in the human sciatic nerve. The majority of these axons are of small diameter (<6μm) and convey information about pain and temperature as well as autonomic functions.

Table 1.1 Classification and conduction velocity of axons in human nerves. After Lloyd (sensory classification) and Erlanger–Gasser (alternative classification)

			Diameter (μm)	Conduction velocity (m/s)	Classi-fication	Alternative classification
Myelinated						
Somatic	Muscle	Afferent	12–21	70–120	Ia, Ib	Aα
			6–12	15–70	II	Aβ
			1–6	3–30	III	Aδ
		Efferent, α and γ motor neurons	6–12	35–75		A
	Cutaneous	Afferent	6–17	15–100	II	Aβ
			1–6	3–30		Aδ
Autonomic preganglionic		Efferent	3	3–15		B
Unmyelinated						
Autonomic postganglionic		Efferent	0.2–1.5	1–2		C
Somatic axons of dorsal root ganglion		Afferent	0.2–1.5	1–2	IV	C

However, this large group is not tested with routine nerve conduction studies, which reflect only activity in large-diameter axons carrying sensory information about proprioception and vibration, plus motor axons conveying commands to the muscles.

Conduction velocity

From an anatomical perspective just two factors determine **conduction velocity**: axon diameter and myelination (see Chapter 2 for further discussion of conduction velocity). In myelinated A fibres, conduction velocity is proportional to diameter, increasing by about 6m/s/μm diameter, whereas unmyelinated fibre conduction velocity is proportional to the square root of the diameter, and increases by about 1.7m/s/μm.

Fastest conducting axons = large diameter + myelinated

Fascicular nerve injury

Nerve fibres are grouped together in fascicles, which usually innervate a common target (Fig. 1.2). Partial nerve lesions are common, and may cause selective damage to fascicles rendered vulnerable by their anatomical arrangement,

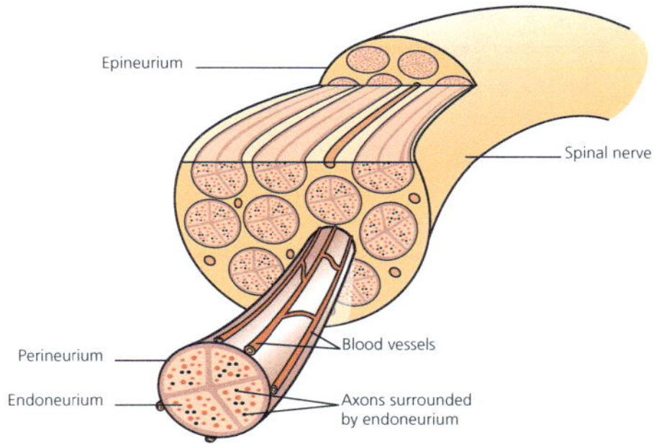

Figure 1.2 Nerve structure: fascicles, endoneurium, and blood supply. Endoneurium surrounds individual axons, perineurium binds each fascicle, and epineurium is the external connective tissue around all the fascicles.

the degree to which they are tethered, their blood supply, the arrangement of their axons and so on. This results in a clinical deficit affecting only part of the territory supplied by that nerve. Examples of partial injury include high sciatic stretch injuries, which commonly damage the peroneal nerve much more than the tibial, or ulnar neuropathies at the elbow, which occasionally affect the fascicle destined for the first dorsal interosseous more than axons supplying the abductor digiti minimi.

Anatomy and the prognosis of nerve injury

The structure of nerves has a crucial bearing on prognosis following nerve injury. Individual axons are surrounded by a connective tissue sheath called endoneurium, the integrity of which determines the likelihood of axon regeneration and eventual clinical recovery after axonal injury (discussed further in Chapter 8).

Neuromuscular Junction

The normal activity of the neuromuscular junction (Fig. 1.3) is described in the following sections, and forms a basis on which to understand specialized neurophysiological tests in disease (considered in Chapter 9).

Activation

1. The action potential depolarizes the nerve terminus, causing presynaptic voltage-gated calcium channels to open, resulting in an influx of Ca^{2+}.
2. The rise in intracellular Ca^{2+} triggers the release of acetylcholine vesicles from the short-term active zone stores, and subsequent discharge of acetylcholine into the synaptic space. A single action potential releases around 60 vesicles, each containing about 6000 molecules of acetylcholine.

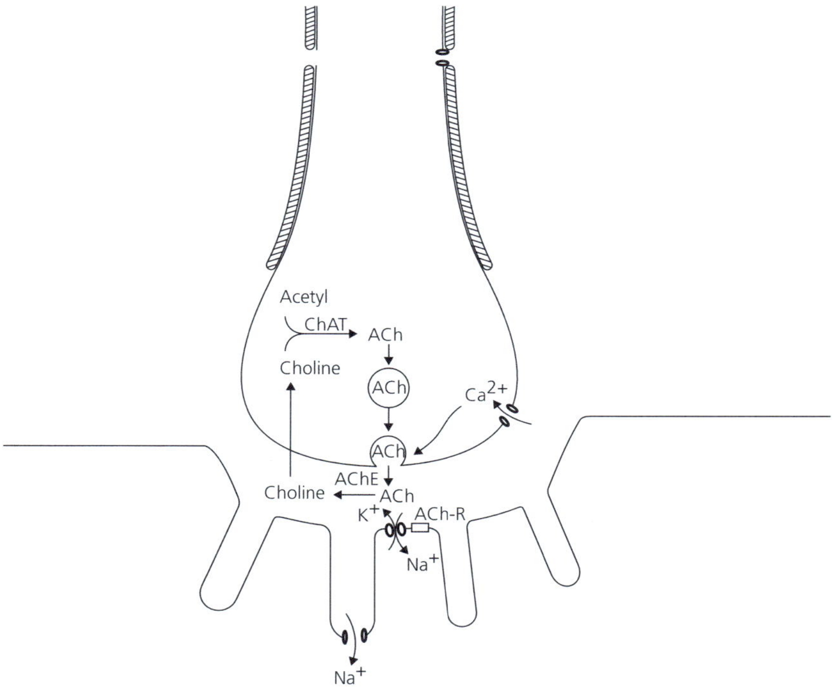

Figure 1.3 The neuromuscular junction.

ACh: acetylcholine, ChAT choline acetyltransferase; AChE: acetylcholinesterase; ACh-R acetylcholine receptor.

3. Acetylcholine attaches to the alpha subunits of the postsynaptic nicotinic acetylcholine receptor, and if both are bound the receptor opens, allowing an influx of Na^+, which generates the **end-plate potential**.
4. Because of the safety factor, the end-plate potential usually comfortably exceeds the threshold for activation of the voltage-gated sodium channels ($Na_v1.4$) in the depth of the synaptic folds, thus a self-propagating action potential is generated in that muscle fibre.

Recovery

1. The acetylcholine receptor closes and releases acetylcholine.
2. Acetylcholine is hydrolysed by acetylcholinesterase to choline and acetate. The choline is taken up by the presynaptic terminus, and acetylcholine resynthesized by choline acetyltransferase, then repackaged into vesicles.

Muscle Anatomy

Intrafusal muscle fibres play a role in monitoring muscle stretch, and receive gamma motor neuron innervation. They are small and non-contractile, and will not be considered further as they are not examined by EMG.

Extrafusal muscle fibres, on the other hand, are contractile, they are supplied by alpha motor neurons, and are the fibre type examined by EMG. Each muscle fibre is a single multinucleate cell approximately 30–100μm in diameter (more like 10μm in neonates) and up to about 12cm in length in adults. There are usually 20–60 muscle fibres per fascicle and several **motor units** contribute to a fascicle (Fig. 1.4). However, muscle fibres of a single motor unit may be distributed over many fascicles, and they may cover a roughly circular cross-sectional region 4–12mm in diameter which, depending on the muscle, may be somewhere in the region of 20–30% of the total muscle cross-sectional area. Fibres from 20–50 motor units share this same volume of muscle. These figures are a rough guide for limb muscles, but the size of both the motor units and muscles varies greatly (see 'The motor unit').

Muscle fibres can be broadly separated into two types according to their physiology and function (see Table 1.2). It should be noted that routine EMG is dominated by activity of type I fibres, which are active during gentle contraction. Because of this the EMG is insensitive to myopathies that selectively affect type II fibres, such as steroid-induced myopathies or muscle wasting associated with chronic disease.

The motor unit

The concept of the motor unit is vital to an understanding of nerve conduction and EMG. This functional unit is comprised of a single anterior horn cell, its axon, and all of the muscle fibres it innervates (Fig. 1.5).

There is great variation in the size of motor units in different muscles of normal human subjects (Table 1.3). The innervation ratio, i.e. the ratio between a motor neuron and the muscle fibres it supplies, is roughly proportional to muscle size. In human laryngeal muscles there may be fewer than ten muscle fibres in a motor unit, whereas in the gastrocnemius, where fine control of movement is not necessary, there may be as many as 1900 muscle fibres per motor unit. There is considerable variation between estimates of innervation ratios depending on the technique used to assess them, histological versus electrical.

In health, the muscle fibres from a single motor unit are interspersed with those from other motor units (shown in Fig. 1.4). If studied in cross-section,

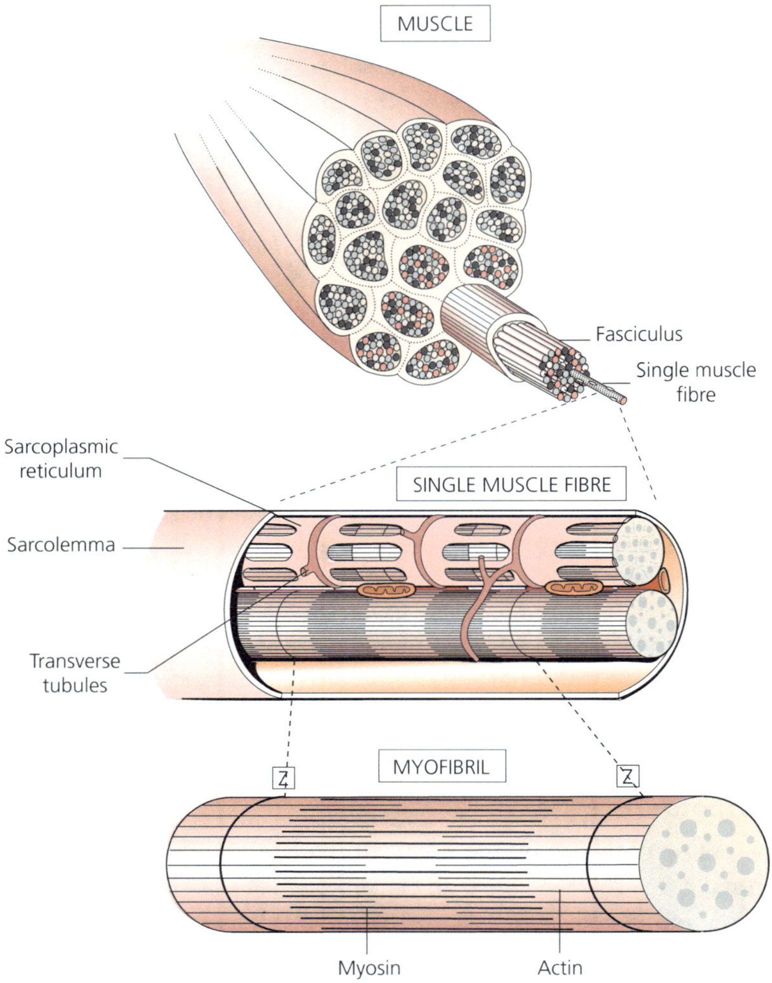

Figure 1.4 Muscle structure, showing the distribution and interspersion of muscle fibres from different motor units. Muscle fibres from a single motor unit shown in red.
Z: z-disk

the area covered by a single motor unit relates to the number of muscle fibres in that motor unit. This changes with disease, and motor unit remodelling after axonal damage results in clusters of muscle fibres supplied by the same axon lying adjacent to one another (discussed further in Chapter 5). Very large motor units develop, in which an abnormally large number of muscle fibres share a common innervation and are dispersed over a wide area.

Table 1.2 EMG and different types of muscle fibre. Note that type I fibres dominate the EMG

	Type I fibre	**Type II fibre (subdivided to fatigable and fatigue-resistant)**
EMG		
Analysed on EMG	Yes predominantly	Not really
Location in muscle	Deep	Superficial
Motor unit size	Small, activate with gentle contraction	Large, activate with strong contraction
Histology and function		
Colour	Red (myoglobin)	White
Contraction time	Slow	Fast
Diameter	Small	Large
Metabolism	Aerobic	Anaerobic glycolysis

Within a motor unit all muscle fibres are either type I or II, not mixed. The type of muscle fibre is determined by the innervating nerve, such that muscle fibres reinnervated after injury become the same type as the remainder of that motor unit, resulting in fibre type grouping. There is some variation in the ratio of the different types of muscle fibre between different muscles, depending on whether the muscle is primarily to maintain posture (type I dominates) or for bursts of forceful contraction (type II).

In general, smaller motor neurons have thinner axons and contact more type I muscle fibres, so are examined well by EMG. On the other hand, some large motor neurons have thick axons and generally innervate type II muscle fibres, forming large motor units that are less well examined with EMG.

Despite the size of some motor units it is important to appreciate that just 5–12 muscle fibres lying within a 0.5mm radius of the needle tip contribute most of the high-voltage spike of the **motor unit action potential** seen during routine **concentric needle** EMG. Although the duration of that potential is influenced by more of the muscle fibres it is clear that the motor unit action potential is only a sample of the activity of a motor unit. If the needle is moved slightly, a different sample of fibres within the same motor unit is made. Furthermore, only a proportion of the total number of motor units is studied, so it is not surprising that patchy pathology can be missed. This is discussed further in Chapters 4–6.

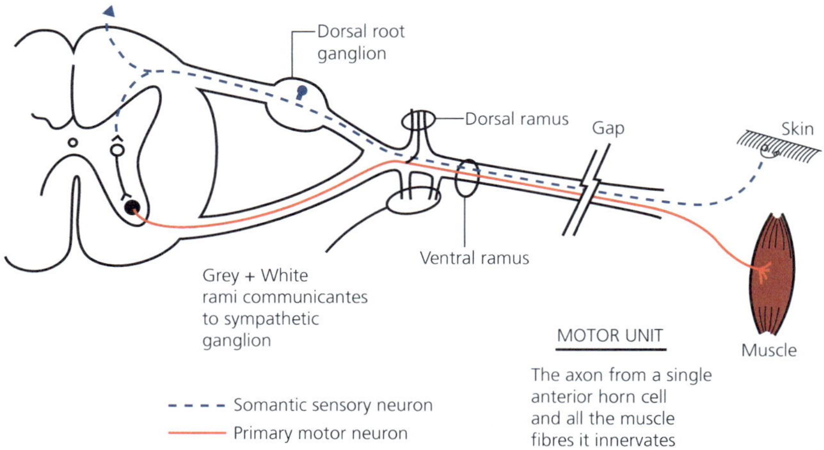

Figure 1.5 The motor unit and peripheral large diameter sensory nerves.
Adapted from *Barr's The Human Nervous System: An Anatomical Viewpoint*, with permission from Lippencott, Williams & Wilkins.

Table 1.3 Motor unit size varies according to muscle. Note that numbers are approximate—some variation relates to the technique used to determine them, histological versus neurophysiological

Muscle	Approximate no. of motor units	Innervation ratio (muscle fibres per motor unit)
Laryngeal	Up to 140	3–25
1st dorsal interosseous	100	100–300
Tibialis anterior	400	300–600
Gastrocnemius	600	400–1900

Muscle contraction

Each muscle fibre is surrounded by a lipid bilayer, the sarcolemma, along which the action potential propagates. The T (transverse) tubules are extensions of the sarcolemma that transmit the action potential through the thickness of the muscle fibre to individual myofibrils. The muscle action potential travels relatively slowly in both directions from the end plate (at below 5m/s, compared to 50m/s in myelinated nerves), and depolarizes the muscle fibre from its resting potential of approximately −80mV.

Depolarization triggers Ca^{2+} release from the sarcoplasmic reticulum, allowing it to bathe the myofibrils and potentiate contraction for approximately 30ms. Ca^{2+} interacts with troponin C, causing a shift of tropomysin which blocks the interaction between actin and myosin in the resting state. Thus contraction is permitted.

The force of muscular contraction depends on two factors: firing rate and number of muscle fibres activated. With minimal contraction one or two small motor neurons will fire, thus activating weak motor units and predominantly type I muscle fibres. Firing rate increases to generate greater force of contraction, and at orderly intervals successively larger motor units are recruited—the final ones to be activated being huge, strong motor units primarily consisting of type II muscle fibres. These principles are discussed further in Chapter 5.

Chapter 2

Principles of Nerve Conduction

Key points

- Stimulation must be supramaximal, the nerve is depolarized beneath the cathode.
- Both active and reference recording electrodes contribute to the final waveform recorded.
- The sensory and motor potentials (SNAP and CMAP) are summed interference patterns of many action potentials.
- The sensory response is recorded over the nerve and is measured in μV, whereas the motor response reflects amplification by the muscle and is measured in mV. Motor nerves are not measured directly.
- The sensory and motor waveforms predominantly reflect large-diameter myelinated axon function, and are insensitive to pathology of small-diameter axons.
- The afferent volley of the H-reflex is carried by large sensory axons, whereas both afferent and efferent volleys of the F-wave travel in motor axons.
- A reduction in limb temperature causes slowing of conduction.
- If motor conduction appears not to make sense, consider an anatomical variation in nerve anatomy.
- There are a number of settings in which nerve conduction and EMG may be very limited or impossible.

This chapter considers the basic principles of routine nerve conduction techniques using surface electrodes. The effects of disease are considered in Chapter 3. An understanding of these basic principles is essential in order to be able to correctly interpret neurophysiological test results, and to spot misleading results and artefacts.

Nerve Stimulation

Stimulation of a nerve is usually performed using a probe held against the skin that has a cathode (negative, usually coloured black) a fixed distance from an **anode** (positive, usually red). Depolarization of the nerve occurs beneath the cathode, and the resulting action potential travels both **orthodromically**, in the usual physiological direction, and **antidromically**, opposite to the physiological direction. Distance is measured from the centre of the cathode in order to calculate conduction velocity.

To ensure correct interpretation and reproducibility of nerve conduction studies, the stimulus delivered must be supramaximal so that all axons are activated. Maximal stimulation is determined by gradually increasing the stimulus intensity (usually the current, but also the pulse duration) until the response no longer increases, then delivering a stimulus about 30% greater than this.

Recording

Recording of sensory and **motor responses** is routinely performed using two surface electrodes (standard electrocardiogram electrodes are sometimes used), with the 'active' referred to the 'reference' electrode. It is important not to think that the reference electrode is inactive or silent, since it plays an important role in shaping the response that is recorded.

In clinical practice, the position of both **recording electrodes** is important. If the recording electrodes are very close together the response recorded will be tend to be small, since there will be less potential difference between the two electrodes as the wave of depolarization (the action potential) passes beneath them. The advantage of having recording electrodes close together is that artefact is minimized since it is likely to affect both electrodes similarly, thus be cancelled when one is referred to the other. On the other hand, if the two electrodes are increasingly widely spaced, the recorded waveform will not continue to increase in **amplitude** beyond a certain point, and the response will tend to be more affected by artefact. Standard recording electrode spacing of about 3cm is used to minimize variability when recording sensory responses.

What is measured?

No matter what the neuromuscular disease, there are generally three key parameters of the sensory or motor response waveform used in routine clinical practice. This makes basic interpretation of nerve conduction studies relatively straightforward.

1. *Velocity.* The initial deflection of the sensory or motor response away from **baseline** is generally used to calculate conduction velocity. It is important to appreciate that this choice of reference point reflects activity in the fastest conducting axons.

Causes of conduction slowing

- **Demyelination.**
- Cold extremities.
- Severe axon loss resulting in loss of fast large-diameter axons.
- Inaccurate measurement, especially small distances across joints.
- Older age, tall patients (minor effects), very young patients.

2. *Amplitude.* Depends on the absolute number of action potentials, and the synchrony of their arrival at the recording electrode. Fewer action potentials or loss of synchrony (termed **temporal dispersion**) will result in a lower amplitude recording, but the two can be distinguished by looking at response duration, which is prolonged with temporal dispersion.

Causes of a low-amplitude compound muscle action potential (CMAP)

Common:

- Motor axon loss.
- Temporal dispersion (CMAP duration is prolonged).
- **Conduction block** between stimulation and recording sites.
- Technical: submaximal stimulation, especially proximal; incorrect electrode placement; oedema.
- Anomalous innervation.

Less common:

- Distal: severe neuromuscular junction pathology, neuromuscular blockade, severe **myopathy.**
- Proximal: severe multilevel motor root or anterior horn cell pathology.

3. *Duration*. Reflects the degree of temporal dispersion, and helps determine whether a loss of amplitude is due to a reduction in the number of action potentials, or the synchrony of their arrival.

Constructive and destructive interference

The sensory nerve action potential, derived from the individual action potentials in many sensory axons, and the CMAP, derived from muscle fibre action potentials, are both summed **interference patterns**. A basic understanding of constructive and **destructive interference** helps understand how these potentials might be affected by neuromuscular disease (Fig. 2.1).

When two identical waveforms are entirely in **phase** the resulting summed waveform will have the same duration, but be twice the amplitude due to **constructive interference**. If, on the other hand, they are asynchronous, for example, they are 180 degrees out of phase, the interference pattern will tend to be of lower amplitude (and longer duration) because of destructive interference.

In reality, both the sensory action potential and the CMAP reflect the summed interference pattern of many action potentials arriving at slightly different times (different phases) because of variation in their conduction times. In addition, the contribution of individual action potentials to the sum is less in those fibres distant from the surface recording electrodes than in those passing directly beneath the electrodes.

When action potentials are more synchronous, the response is high amplitude and short duration, and when less synchronous, for example, with patchy demyelination causing differences in conduction velocity, the amplitude is low and the duration long. In clinical neurophysiology the term *temporal*

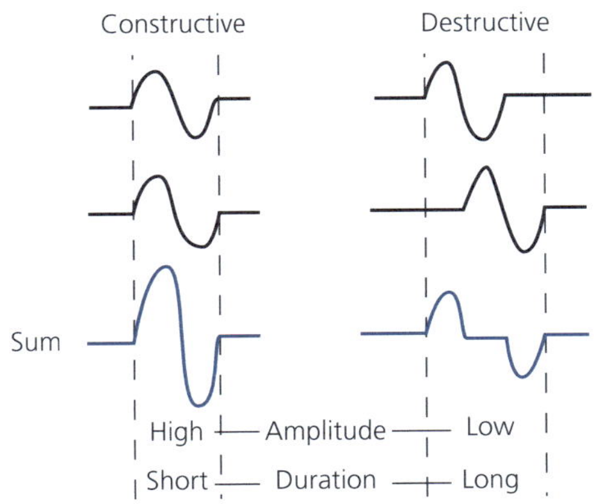

Figure 2.1 Constructive and destructive interference.

dispersion is used to describe the loss of synchrony of action potentials resulting in a low-amplitude, long-duration compound potential. This is considered further in Chapter 3.

Large-diameter axons are recorded in clinical practice

It is important to appreciate that routine nerve conduction studies reflect activity in large-diameter axons. Experimental studies have shown that the waveform recorded after electrical stimulation of a nerve consists of a number of peaks corresponding to the different conduction velocities of the constituent axons—faster if broader and myelinated, thus seen earlier in the recorded waveform (Fig. 2.2).

During routine clinical recordings made with surface electrodes, many of the small late peaks are lost or unreliable, leaving only the high-amplitude earlier peak to be measured as discussed later in this chapter. Conduction velocity is routinely measured with reference to the onset of the motor or sensory response, so is determined by the fast, broad, myelinated fibres.

This bias towards measurement of large-diameter nerve fibres has two important implications for the interpretation of nerve conduction studies. Firstly, pathology selectively affecting small-diameter fibres will be completely missed, which is a serious omission since the majority of human peripheral

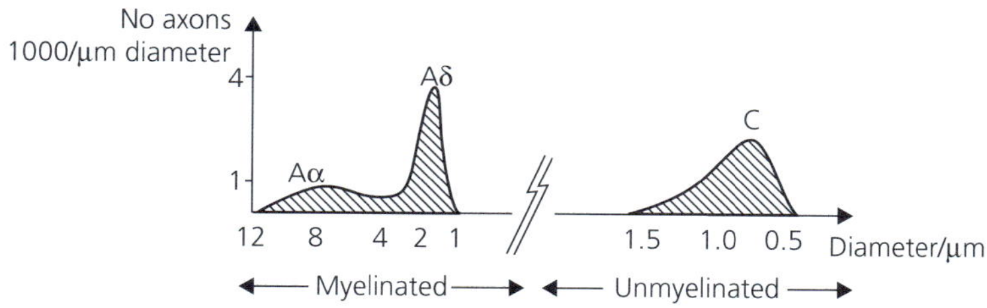

Figure 2.2 Sensory compound action potential waveform, measured *in vitro* (top panel). Late peaks reflect slow-conducting fibres that are narrow diameter or unmyelinated. They are not detected in routine clinical studies. In clinical practice the Aα peak is measured. This corresponds to a small number of large diameter axons.

nerve axons have a narrow diameter of <6μm. Fortunately, selective **small-fibre** neuropathies can usually be identified by their distinct clinical presentation (with, for example, burning pain and altered temperature sensibility), and they can be tested for in a range of different ways beyond the scope of this book. Secondly, when there is severe axonal pathology there will tend to be a reduction in the measured conduction velocity because of loss of very fast conducting fibres. This is not to be confused with the conduction slowing typical of demyelinating neuropathies and is discussed further in Chapter 3.

Sensory Nerve Action Potential (SNAP)

The **compound sensory nerve action potential** recorded by surface electrodes is the sum of individual action potentials in many large-diameter sensory axons.

Isolation

There are many purely sensory peripheral nerves amenable to direct stimulation and recording, but the neurophysiologist often needs to isolate the sensory component of mixed nerves. One way is by selective distal stimulation of sensory fibres where they run separately from motor fibres. Recording is made proximally, but is not affected by the motor fibres at this level since they are not stimulated. An example would be stimulation of pure sensory median nerves in the finger, recording orthodromic transmission proximally at the wrist where the nerve also contains unstimulated motor axons. The alternative approach is proximal stimulation of mixed sensory and motor fibres with distal recording of the pure sensory response beyond the point at which motor axons have separated. An example is mixed median nerve stimulation at the wrist, with recording of a purely sensory response from digital nerves. The two techniques give slightly different amplitude responses, so it is important to know which is used.

Site of the recording electrodes

Both active and reference electrodes are placed on the skin directly overlying the nerve. Given the expected duration of the compound depolarization waveform (1–2msec) and velocity with which it travels (about 50m/s), an interelectrode distance of about 3cm is commonly used to maximize amplitude since one electrode is likely to record the peak whilst the other records the trough of the travelling wave.

Waveform

See Fig. 2.3.

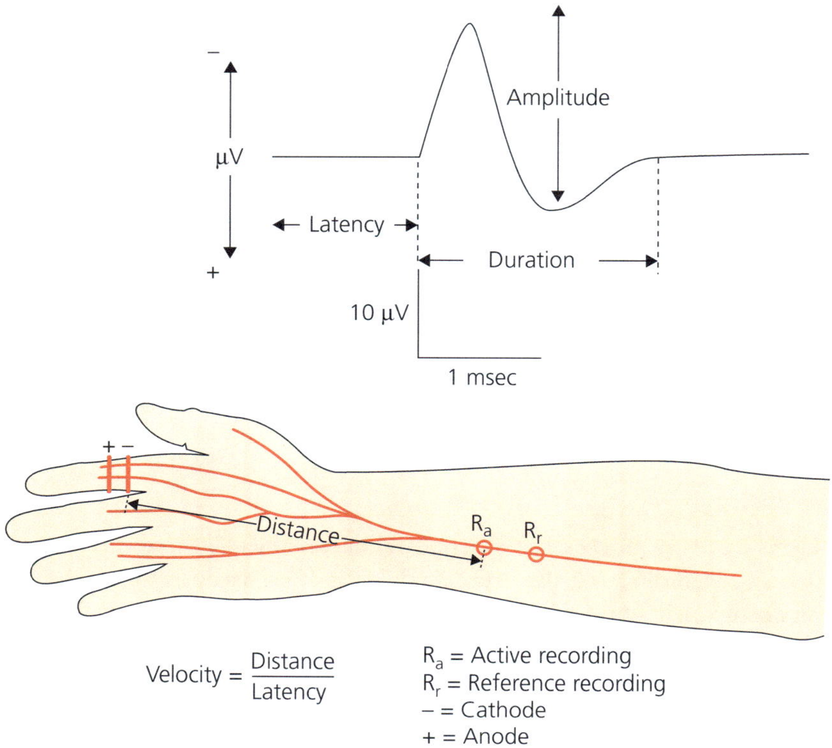

Figure 2.3 Measurement of the compound sensory nerve action potential (SNAP). Note the neurophysiological convention that upwards deflection is negative. Unfortunately there is not international uniformity of measurement parameters. Some laboratories will record orthodromic sensory responses measuring latency to initial waveform deflection from baseline, and peak-to-peak measurement for amplitude (shown in the figure). Others will record antidromic responses, latency to the negative peak and use baseline to negative peak amplitude measurements.

Adapted from Preston and Shapiro. *Electromyography and Neuromuscular Disorders*. Copyright (2005), with permission from Elsevier, and from Liveson and Ma. *Laboratory Reference for Clinical Neurophysiology*. © Oxford University Press, 1999.

Units

Measured in μV (compare with mV for the CMAP).

Velocity

The distance between the centre of the stimulating cathode and the active recording electrode is divided by the time taken to travel between the two.

Table 2.1 Comparison of sensory and motor nerve conduction measurements

	Sensory, SNAP	Motor, CMAP
Activity recorded	Nerve	Muscle
Amplitude	μV, peak to trough (check local practice)	mV, negative peak only
Duration	1–2ms	5–15ms
Velocity	Single site stimulation	Requires two sites of stimulation

Compound Muscle Action Potential (CMAP)

The **CMAP** is a compound surface potential reflecting the sum of individual action potentials in many muscle fibres. It is therefore not a direct recording of the motor nerves, but of the muscles they activate. It differs in many ways from the sensory nerve action potential (see Table 2.1). It is important to keep in mind that the CMAP is a recording of electrical activity, and not of strength of muscle contraction. It is generally correct that a normal CMAP corresponds to the muscle being strong, but this is not the case if there is proximal conduction block, and would not be the case if there was failure of electromechanical coupling within muscle fibres.

Isolation

The motor component of peripheral nerves is assessed indirectly, by recording the summed action potentials of muscle fibres that it innervates (not the mechanical twitch). Muscle electrical activity is a marker of motor nerve activity, intimately connected by the neuromuscular junction. This indirect recording of motor nerve activity has a number of important consequences:

1. The CMAP may be small due to failure of neuromuscular transmission or pathology of the muscle, so does not necessarily imply abnormality of the motor nerve.
2. Responses are amplified. CMAPs are measured in mV, compared to sensory and **mixed nerve** response amplitudes measured in μV.
3. The neuromuscular junction and muscle contribute to a considerable time lag between depolarization at the distal nerve and subsequent recording of the CMAP. This means motor **nerve conduction velocity** cannot be calculated in the same way as sensory nerves, and requires two sites of stimulation.

Site of the recording electrodes

The **active electrode** is placed over the end-plate region, which in most muscles is at its centre. This ensures an initial negative (upwards) deflection from baseline since the muscle action potential originates under the active electrode. If the electrode is incorrectly sited, or a neighbouring muscle inadvertently stimulated, the initial CMAP deflection is likely to be positive (downwards), implying initial muscle activation is distant from the active electrode, and suggesting technique should be checked. The reference electrode is usually sited on the distal tendon of the muscle since this is relatively electrically silent, yet near enough that it tends to be affected by similar noise to the active electrode. Noise will therefore be minimized in the final output since this is the potential difference between active and reference electrodes.

Waveform

See Fig. 2.4.

Units

Measured in mV (compare with μV for sensory nerve responses).

Velocity

The muscle is stimulated from two different points along the nerve, and the distance between the two is divided by the difference in onset **latency** of the CMAPs. This removes the time interval between the distal point of stimulation and CMAP onset with the assumption that the delay in neuromuscular transmission remains the same in the two situations (valid for routine clinical use).

Mixed Nerve Studies

Mixed sensory and motor nerves are tested in an analogous way to the pure sensory studies already described, but with both the stimulation and recording points over the nerve where it carries mixed fibres. The response recorded is influenced by both sensory and motor axons, although in most situations it is dominated by large-diameter sensory fibres. The conduction velocity is determined by the largest and fastest of all human nerve fibres, the 1a muscle afferents (see Chapter 1) which are not recorded in pure sensory or motor studies, thus the mixed nerve action potential often has the fastest conduction velocity of all nerves studied.

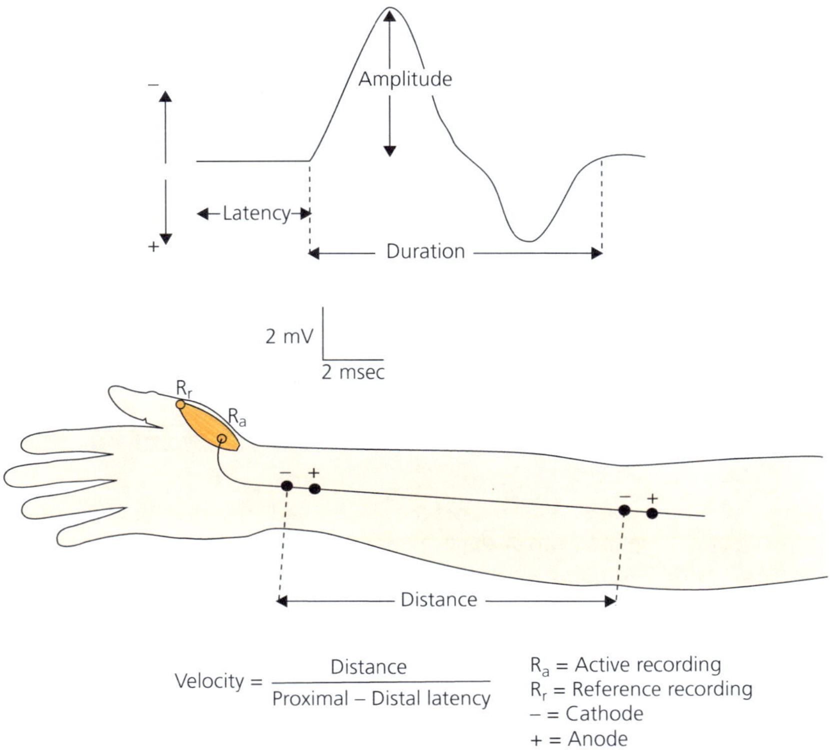

Figure 2.4 Measurement of the compound muscle action potential (CMAP). Note the neurophysiological convention that upwards deflection is negative. Latency is measured to the initial waveform deflection from baseline, and amplitude is from baseline to negative peak (check local practice).

Adapted from Liveson, J. and Ma, D. *Laboratory Reference for Clinical Neurophysiology.* © Oxford University Press, 1999.

Longer Latency Responses

F-waves

Following motor nerve stimulation there is a direct muscle response, known as the **M-wave** (the routine CMAP), followed by a small amplitude response which occurs considerably later, the **F-wave**. The F-wave is non-physiological, and results from electrical nerve stimulation causing an antidromically conducted action potential in the motor axon which, on arrival at the spinal cord, causes a proportion of the anterior horn cells at that level to fire again. Note that, in contrast to the H-reflex, both the afferent and efferent action potentials are carried in the motor axon, with no involvement of sensory axons (see Fig 2.5).

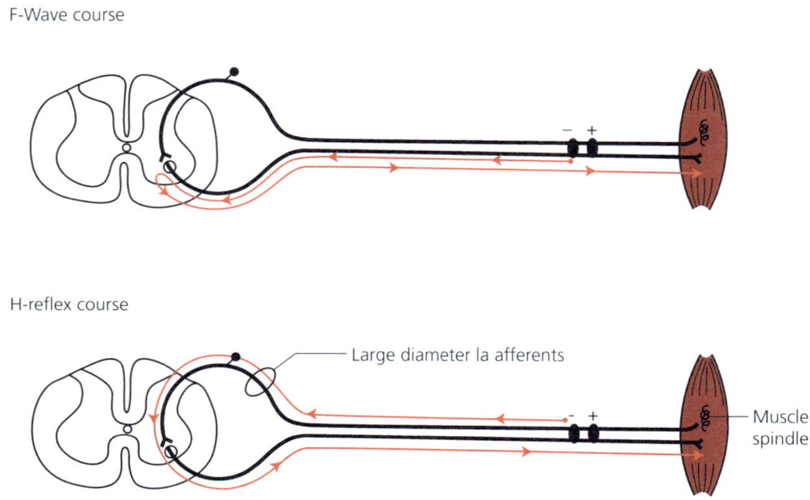

Figure 2.5 F-wave versus H-reflex. Both the afferent and efferent limbs of the F-wave response pass along the axons of alpha motor neurons. In contrast the afferent course of the H-reflex travels via large diameter 1a sensory axons, and the efferent course is along alpha motor neurons.

With repeated nerve stimulation, normal F-waves show slight variation, both in amplitude and latency, thus it is common practice to measure a series of responses (at least ten) to determine minimum latency (the most commonly used parameter in clinical practice), persistence, or other measurements. F-waves reflect conduction along the entire length of the peripheral nerve, and show good test–retest reproducibility. They might seem an excellent way of testing the relatively inaccessible proximal portions of the nerve and its roots. However, their sensitivity is limited since they travel via a number of motor roots, not just one, so may remain relatively unaffected despite severe lesions to some of these roots provided adjacent ones are unaffected.

H-reflex

The H-reflex is the neurophysiological equivalent of the deep tendon reflex (albeit with the muscle spindle bypassed), so it is absent when the corresponding reflex cannot be obtained. Using a long-duration stimulus and very gradual increments in intensity, there is initial preferential activation of large-diameter 1a afferents. These synapse to alpha motor neurons in the spinal cord, which fire and activate the muscle, from where the **H-wave** can be recorded. As stimulus intensity is increased, the direct short-latency M-wave becomes visible, the H-wave disappears, and the F-wave can be seen.

Although H-reflexes can be obtained from a number of sites the most frequently used is recorded form the soleus following stimulation of the tibial nerve in the popliteal fossa. The soleus H-reflex predominantly traverses the S1 root, and is of some help in localizing focal proximal lesions in this region.

Undesired Sources of Variability

The interpretation of results from the neurophysiological examination depends on their reproducibility and the range of normal values. Of course one potential source of variability is technique, but there are other physiological and anatomical factors. This is particularly true for nerve conduction studies, considered next, although there are more subtle changes in EMG too.

Physiological

Temperature has a marked effect on nerve and muscle conduction. For every degree below 32°C there is approximately 1–2m/s slowing in motor and sensory conduction velocity, although the effect is probably not linear. Furthermore, sensory nerve and CMAP amplitudes tend to increase in the cold. It is therefore important to correct limb temperature to 32°C wherever possible, but this takes a few minutes since it is nerve temperature, not that of the skin, which is important. A less satisfactory solution is to record skin temperature, and make allowance when interpreting results.

Age affects nerves, with conduction velocity tending to decrease by up to 1–2m/s for every decade above 60 years old, although there is variation between subjects. In addition, sensory, and to a lesser extent motor, response amplitudes may decrease with age, but again there is considerable intersubject variation. For example, for patients over 70 years old it is relatively common to be unable to record a sural nerve sensory response, or for the extensor digitorum brevis CMAP to be very small, so these findings should not necessarily be considered pathological.

Although there is an effect of height (taller people tend to have slower peripheral conduction velocities) and sex these effects are relatively small.

Anatomical

There are relatively common variants in nerve anatomy, in which a proportion of axons travel in a different nerve to that expected for some of their course. These often come to light during nerve conduction studies, and unless understood they can compromise the interpretation of results. Usually there are characteristic clues, such as appearance of an initial

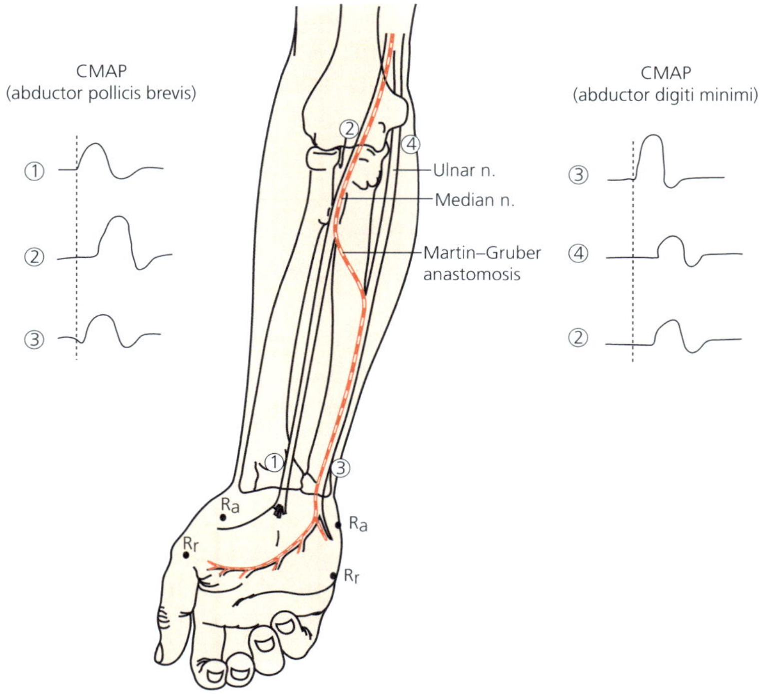

Figure 2.6 One example of a Martin–Gruber anastomosis. Note that when recording a CMAP from abductor digiti minimi this type of anastomosis results in a pseudo conduction block pattern: the CMAP following stimulation over the ulnar nerve at site 4 is small. However, the muscle will not be weak, and the missing axons are revealed by stimulation over the median nerve in the antecubital fossa, site 2.

positive CMAP deflection or greater amplitude with proximal versus distal stimulation.

The most common is a Martin–Gruber anastomosis, where there is communication between the median and ulnar nerves in the forearm (Fig. 2.6). A proportion of axons that run proximally in the median nerve cross to run distally with the ulnar nerve, eventually innervating any of the following ulnar innervated muscles: the abductor digiti minimi, the first dorsal interosseous or the thenar muscles (adductor pollicis, deep head of flexor pollicis brevis). Depending on the exact pattern of innervation these anomalies may be detected in routine ulnar nerve conduction studies as pseudo-conduction block, with reduced amplitude responses following both below- and above-elbow stimulation in comparison to wrist stimulation (yet, of course, no weakness, therefore no clinical suspicion of motor conduction block). If the crossed fibres supply thenar muscles, median nerve stimulation at the wrist may activate only the usual axons in the nerve at that point destined for the abductor pollicis brevis muscle. However, median nerve stimulation at the elbow activates many more nerve fibres to thenar muscles, some being the crossed fibres destined for ulnar innervated thenar muscles, thus eliciting a larger CMAP.

Another common anatomical variant involves the extensor digitorum brevis, usually supplied by the deep peroneal nerve. In some people a proportion of axons travel via the superficial peroneal nerve, and then branch off this nerve in an accessory deep peroneal nerve to innervate the muscle. In this instance there is a smaller CMAP elicited from the extensor digitorum brevis with distal compared to proximal stimulation of the deep peroneal nerve. The 'lost' axons are identified by stimulation of the accessory nerve behind the lateral malleolus.

Practical Issues

It is not uncommon for neurophysiological laboratories to be referred patients in whom testing is unsuitable, or is likely to provide little useful information, due to foreseeable problems. Understanding some of these obstacles should make testing safer and avoid wasted appointments or disappointment if testing is limited.

Restrictions to nerve conduction testing

1. Oedema or severe obesity may make it impossible to record surface responses, particularly distal lower limb responses (and may also limit needle EMG).
2. Bandages and casts are likely to impede either recording or stimulation, and adhesive electrodes cannot be applied to areas of broken skin.
3. Caution must be taken if a patient has a pacemaker or implantable cardiac defibrillator. Repetitive stimulation and proximal upper limb studies are particular concerns.

Restrictions to needle EMG

1. Anticoagulation—although not necessarily an absolute contraindication, the electromyographer should be informed and the international normalization ratio known. Muscles in tight fascial spaces are usually avoided.
2. Bleeding disorders, particularly haemophilia or if thrombocytopenia $<30{,}000/mm^3$.
3. Cellulitis or other surface skin infection.
4. Lymphoedema is a relative contraindication.

Overall limiting factors

1. Patient cooperation with the test: children, cognitive impairment.
2. Timing of neurophysiological examination in relation to injury. Depends on the referral question—see Chapter 8.

Chapter 3

Nerve Conduction in Disease

Key points

- Axon loss causes a reduction in response amplitude, whereas demyelination commonly results in conduction slowing.
- Demyelination may cause conduction block or temporal dispersion. Both reduce response amplitude, but temporal dispersion also prolongs the duration of the response.
- Conduction velocity can be reduced to about 70% of the lower limit of normal as a result of very severe axon loss without demyelination.
- The degree of conduction slowing is in proportion to axon loss, so if the CMAP amplitude is normal even mild slowing can suggest demyelination.
- Amplitude and area of responses can help quantify axon loss.
- Homogeneous severe demyelination is suggestive of a hereditary demyelinating neuropathy, whereas patchy findings are more suggestive of an inflammatory aetiology.
- Conduction block and axon loss cause muscle weakness, but conduction slowing alone does not.
- If there is no muscle weakness do not trust nerve conduction results that appear suggestive of motor conduction block.
- Conduction block is due to dysfunction of the nodes of Ranvier causing failure of action potential propagation. Sometimes it recovers quickly.
- Conduction block cannot be reliably diagnosed when there is temporal dispersion or when response amplitudes are small.

Basic assessment of nerve pathology using conduction studies is relatively straightforward since there are just two key pathologies: axon loss and demyelination. Furthermore, most abnormalities of the waveforms recorded can be described by three parameters: velocity of propagation, amplitude, and duration. Axon loss will result in a reduction in the amplitude of the response recorded, and demyelination will generally cause slowing of conduction.

Whilst these principles are true, there is a degree of complication since severe axon loss will also result in a slight decrease in the measured conduction velocity. Also, demyelination can result in a reduction in response amplitude due to temporal dispersion or conduction block, so loss of response amplitude does not always imply axonal pathology. Furthermore, it is common to find mixed pathology, for example, secondary axon loss with primarily demyelinating pathology. The distinction of axonal versus demyelinating pathology is important since it has implications for diagnosis, prognosis, and treatment.

This chapter will consider the basic principles of nerve conduction when there is pathology affecting the nerves, not special tests such as those of the neuromuscular junction that are reviewed in Chapter 9. In addition, this chapter will not consider how to localize pathology since this is covered in Chapter 7.

Axon Loss

If there is motor axon loss there are fewer muscle fibres activated, and the sum of all their action potentials, the CMAP, is of lower amplitude and smaller area

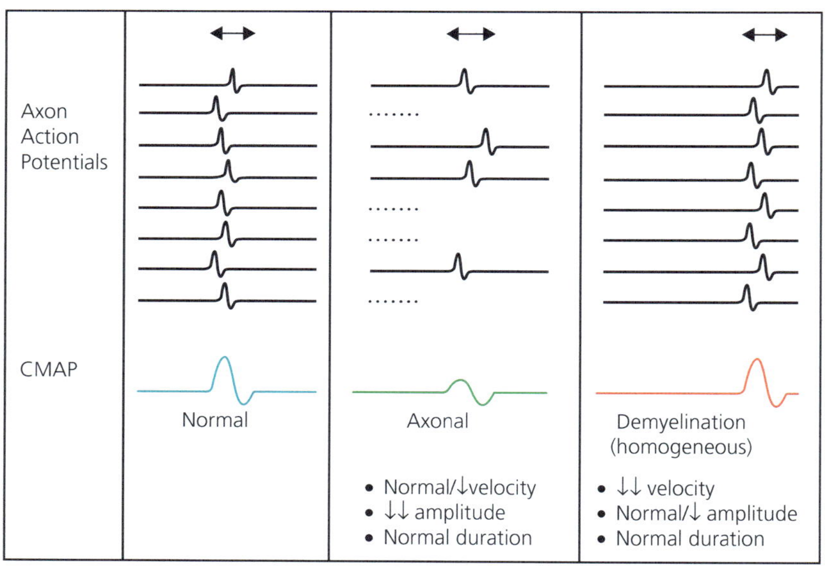

Figure 3.1 Nerve conduction with axonal versus demyelinating pathology. Compound muscle action potential (CMAP)–the sum of individual muscle fibre action potentials. With axon loss the summed amplitude is small, and with demyelination the nerve conduction velocity is usually slowed.

(measured beneath the negative, upward, phase of the CMAP. See Fig 3.1). The same principle holds for sensory studies, where loss of axons reduces response amplitude and area.

In a pure axonal lesion the conduction velocity of those motor axons that remain intact is unaffected. As a result, provided there is relatively mild axon loss, the conduction velocity will still be in the normal range or only minimally reduced.

However, when there is severe axon loss, resulting in a CMAP amplitude less than about 25% of the lower limit of normal, there tends to be a reduction in the range of nerve diameters that contribute to the small response recorded by the surface electrodes (Fig 3.2). Furthermore, sometimes the axon loss preferentially affects large-diameter fibres. In either case the result is that conduction velocity is reduced since it is conventionally measured to the initial deflection of the CMAP from baseline, which is determined by the fastest conducting motor axons.

In clinical practice it is generally accepted that severe axon loss, where the CMAP amplitude is below 25% of the lower limit of normal, may result in a reduction of conduction velocity to about 70–75% of the lower limit of normal. In this setting the mild reduction of conduction velocity does not imply additional demyelination. However, slowing beyond this cannot purely relate to severe loss of large-diameter axons, even with a small CMAP, and suggests demyelination.

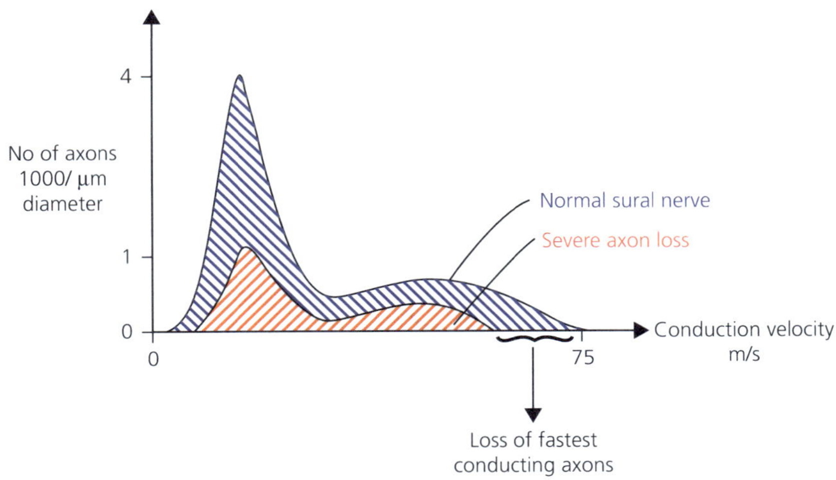

Figure 3.2 Distribution of nerve fibre conduction velocities. Severe axon loss results in loss of the fastest conducting axons, and therefore a small reduction in measured conduction velocity.

The expected reduction in conduction velocity is in proportion to the degree of loss of CMAP amplitude. In other words, mild axon loss, with a slight reduction in CMAP, is not sufficient to explain a reduction in conduction velocity to 70% of normal, suggesting that in this setting there is also demyelination.

Quantification of the amount of axonal pathology may be desirable for prognosis and determining the efficacy of treatment. EMG is a sensitive way of detecting motor axon loss, but generally poor at quantifying it, and of course it is insensitive to sensory axon pathology. On the other hand, changes in the CMAP or sensory response amplitude and area, although less sensitive, provide better estimates of the amount of axon loss and, within the limits of reproducibility, can detect change if repeated over time (see Chapter 7).

Demyelination

Homogeneous demyelination

Some hereditary neuropathies, such as type 1 Charcot–Marie–Tooth (CMT) disease, tend to cause similar severity demyelination of different axons within a nerve, as well as between nerves. Thus, although the individual action potentials travel much more slowly than usual (in CMT 1 often below 20m/s, compared to a normal speed of about 50m/s), the volley of action potentials in different axons remains relatively well synchronized. Although there is inevitably slight loss of synchrony following proximal stimulation, termed temporal dispersion (see 'Temporal dispersion' section), it is relatively mild, thus the normal CMAP morphology is quite well preserved despite the markedly slow conduction velocity (see Fig. 3.1). This should be contrasted with non-homogeneous demyelination causing temporal dispersion, discussed later.

The finding of homogeneous very slow conduction velocities (<50% of normal) without conduction block or temporal dispersion is characteristic of inherited demyelinating neuropathies. Conduction slowing alone does not cause weakness, but there is usually secondary axon loss, even in the inherited demyelinating neuropathies, and over time this increasingly contributes to disability.

Although characteristic, it is not inevitable that demyelination is very severe or entirely homogeneous in the hereditary demyelinating neuropathies. There are 'intermediate' forms of CMT disease, for example, the X-linked form caused by mutations in the protein connexin-32, in which upper limb motor conduction velocities are often in the 30's (m/s) in men and the 40's in women. Furthermore, there are reports of conduction block and temporal dispersion in these patients. These findings are unusual, but significant. Generally, the clinical rule of thumb is that patchy demyelination suggests an acquired inflammatory aetiology, such as chronic inflammatory demyelinating polyneuropathy. However, in patients who remain steadfastly refractory to treatment, it is worth considering testing for atypical hereditary neuropathies such as CMT-X.

Conduction block

Conduction block is caused by dysfunction of the nodes of Ranvier due to a particular type of focal damage to myelin, or dysfunction of the membrane ion channels. The type of myelin pathology is different to that seen in hereditary neuropathies, and presents clinically with focal weakness if motor axons are affected, or numbness if sensory axons are blocked. Unlike the weakness caused by axon loss, there is no muscle wasting.

Although conduction block is generally discussed as a type of 'demyelination', the structural abnormalities of the ensheathing myelin are subtle, if present at all, and there is no loss of Schwann cells. Because the problem is one of function more than structure it is sometimes termed 'dysmyelination' rather than demyelination. The distinction is not merely semantic—conduction block frequently resolves faster than would be expected if complete remyelination were necessary.

If conduction block is suspected, the best way of proving it neurophysiologically is by studying a nerve that supplies a weak, but not wasted, muscle. When the nerve is stimulated below the level of block the resulting CMAP is of normal size and morphology, and conduction velocity is normal. However, stimulation above the site of block results in a small CMAP (provided the block is partial, not complete) because many action potentials fail to propagate through the site of block, so cannot excite their respective muscle fibres (Figs 3.3 and 3.4). Conduction velocity across the region of block is often slightly reduced.

It is very important to determine whether there really is true conduction block since it is likely to imply a particular prognosis and specific treatment. A CMAP may be reduced in amplitude following proximal versus distal stimulation (giving apparent partial motor conduction block) for a number of other reasons, most commonly submaximal proximal stimulation or temporal dispersion. Usually proof that this apparent block is not real comes from clinical examination—muscle strength is maintained. There are published criteria for 'probable' and 'definite' conduction block which specify the reduction in CMAP amplitude and area required over particular nerve segments, and the amount of temporal dispersion acceptable.

Conduction block is more reliably detected in some nerves than others. For example, ulnar nerve motor conduction studies are easily performed and reproducible, making detection easy provided the examiner is aware of the

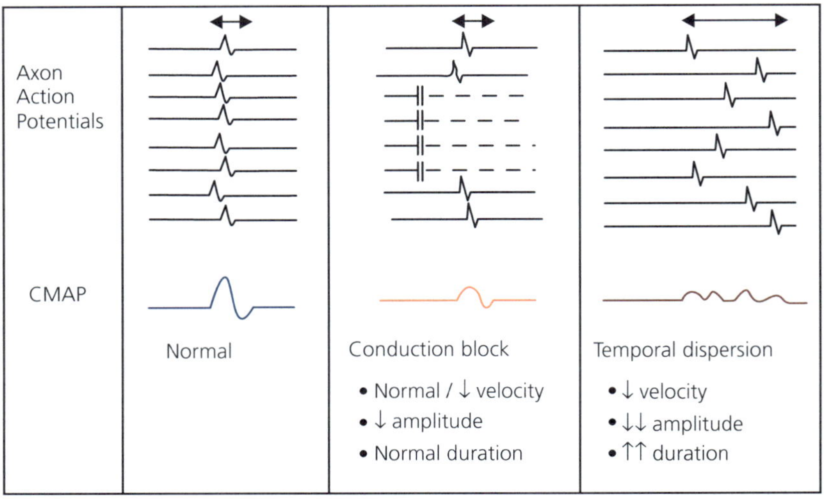

Figure 3.3 Nerve conduction studies with conduction block versus temporal dispersion. Stimulation above the site of partial conduction block results in a low amplitude but normal duration CMAP. With temporal dispersion the amplitude is also reduced, but the duration of the response is prolonged.

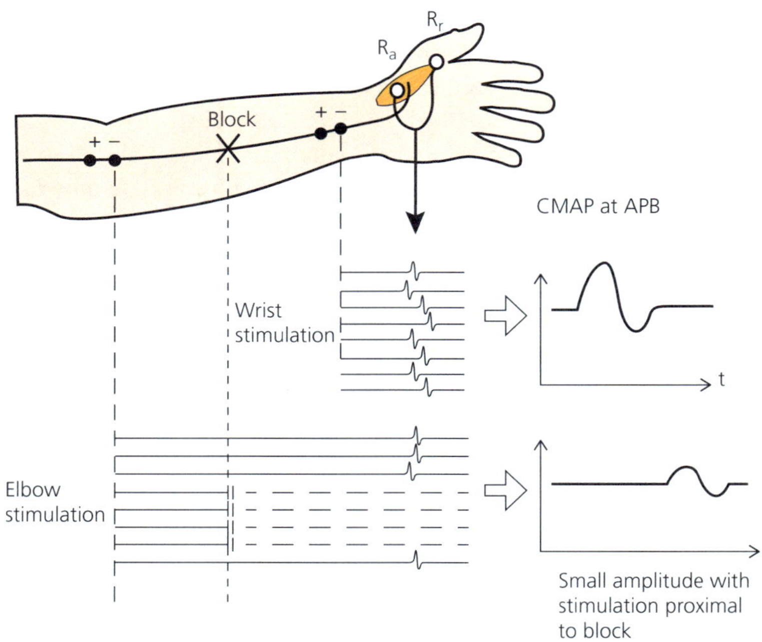

Figure 3.4 Median nerve partial motor conduction block in the forearm.

APB: abductor pollicis brevis

effect of a Martin–Gruber anastomosis (Fig. 2.6). On the other hand, tibial nerve motor studies are less reliable since the nerve may be difficult to stimulate supramaximally at the popliteal fossa, resulting in a small CMAP even in the absence of block. Conduction block, detected by a loss of amplitude and area of the CMAP, cannot be diagnosed in the presence of severe temporal dispersion (see 'Temporal dispersion' section) because this also results in a reduction in amplitude.

Is there really conduction block?

1. *Is the muscle weak?* Significant motor conduction block will cause weakness, so lack of weakness suggests a technical problem or anomalous innervation. Sensory conduction block results in a patch of numbness.
2. *Is there temporal dispersion?* If the CMAP duration is very prolonged with proximal stimulation compared to distal this is termed temporal dispersion, and conduction block is not proven.
3. *How big is the distal CMAP?* Conduction block cannot be reliably diagnosed if the CMAP is very small with distal stimulation, since a further decrease with proximal stimulation is not reliably detected.
4. *How robust is the finding for that nerve?* A small drop in amplitude with proximal stimulation is significant in some, but not all nerves.

Temporal dispersion

If a demyelinating process is patchy, affecting axons to different degrees, the result is greater heterogeneity of conduction velocities and a loss of synchrony of individual action potentials arriving at the recording electrodes. The summed surface interference pattern (the CMAP or SNAP) is therefore abnormally prolonged, termed 'temporal dispersion' (Fig. 3.3).

In general, when there is temporal dispersion without axon loss or conduction block, the CMAP amplitude is reduced but there is little loss of area. However, the loss of synchrony of action potentials may result in a slight increase in destructive interference between individual action potentials, the result being a small decrease in area of the CMAP with proximal stimulation compared to distal (see Chapter 2 for more discussion of interference).

It is useful to contrast conduction block and temporal dispersion. In the former, the CMAP with proximal stimulation tends to remain of short duration yet the amplitude and area are reduced. In the latter, the CMAP duration is prolonged, the amplitude reduced, and the area unchanged or only slightly reduced. In some situations an intermediate result is recorded, where amplitude and area are both moderately reduced and duration moderately prolonged. In this instance, or when distal CMAP amplitudes are small, it can be difficult to determine the relative contribution of conduction block and temporal dispersion, and arbitrary guidelines have been set for research and clinical use. It is always worth considering whether the recorded waveform could reflect temporal dispersion rather than conduction block.

When a CMAP is small due to temporal dispersion or conduction block, EMG assessment of the affected muscle may be helpful in determining whether there is additional axon loss. If present, axon loss may be contributing significantly to weakness, and depending on the clinical setting this may suggest a limited response to treatment, or predict a slower recovery.

Other Conditions May Affect Nerve Conduction Responses

As already described, the main types of pathology that affect nerve conduction are axon loss and demyelination, the latter including homogeneous forms as well as conduction block and temporal dispersion. Pathology at certain sites in the peripheral nervous system typically has no effect on nerve conduction, but when it is severe may cause a reduction in the CMAP amplitude, leaving other conduction parameters unaffected. It is mentioned here for completeness and considered further in Chapter 6, since the diagnosis relies on understanding EMG findings.

Neuromuscular junction pathology has no effect on sensory conduction, but can affect the CMAP amplitude. Severe myasthenia gravis or Lambert–Eaton myasthenic syndrome can result in small CMAPs when failure of neuromuscular transmission results in severe weakness. In both settings the CMAP is reduced because the failure of neuromuscular transmission results in reduced activation of muscle fibres. Both may be diagnosed with special neurophysiological tests, and are considered further in Chapter 9. Severe myopathies can also result in low-amplitude CMAPs because of a decrease in the number of excitable muscle fibres. In this case EMG can usually distinguish denervation due to axon loss from a myopathic cause of small CMAPs.

Proximal pathology, at either the nerve root or anterior horn cell, will likewise typically not be detected by peripheral nerve conduction studies. However, with severe multilevel disease the CMAP may be reduced without any other change in peripheral nerve conduction. Again, EMG helps make the diagnosis and will be discussed further in Chapter 6.

Chapter 4

Anatomy and the Normal EMG

Key points

- Needle movement and variation in the force of muscle contraction are essential in order to study an adequate sample of the motor units in a muscle.
- The motor unit action potential only reflects activity in a fraction of the tens or hundreds of muscle fibres in a motor unit.
- Using a standard concentric EMG needle, the amplitude of the motor unit action potential is determined by about 5–12 muscle fibres within about 0.5mm radius of the needle tip. It is greatly affected by even small movements of the needle.
- Duration of the motor unit action potential is determined by muscle fibres within about 2mm radius of the needle tip, and is less susceptible to slight movement of the needle.
- During EMG examination, the electromyographer must pay particular attention to the following four parameters: spontaneous activity, motor unit action potential morphology, recruitment pattern, and interference pattern.
- The EMG is sensitive to type I muscle fibre pathology, but relatively insensitive to isolated type II muscle fibre disease since these fibres tend to be grouped in large motor units which recruit late (with strong contraction) into an already busy EMG screen.

Anatomy and the EMG Needle

A standard 26-gauge concentric EMG needle has a recording surface of approximately 0.08mm^2, and records changes in electrical potential in a hemisphere up to a 1–2mm radius from its bevelled recording surface. Monopolar EMG needles, favoured by some electrophysiologists because they are cheaper and potentially

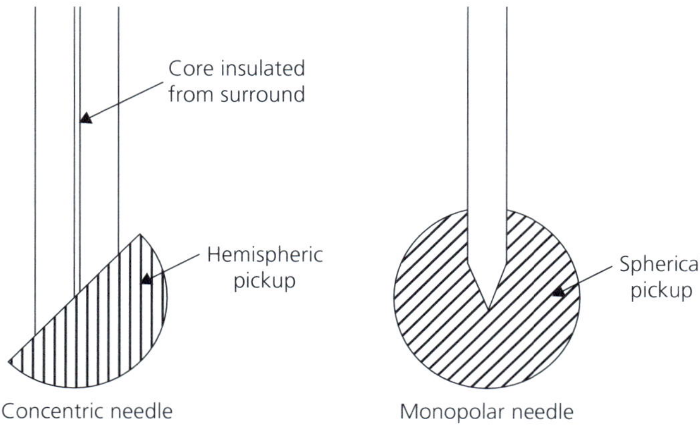

Figure 4.1 Recording volumes of concentric and monopolar EMG needles.

less uncomfortable for the patient, record from a spherical volume a couple of millimetres in radius around the needle tip (Fig. 4.1). Although the potentials recorded with the two needle types are subtly different, the principles of interpretation remain the same, so they will not be considered separately.

The muscle fibres belonging to a single motor unit cover a relatively wide cross-sectional area compared to the recording area of the EMG needle. They are widely spaced, and intermixed with fibres from other motor units (reviewed in Chapter 1). If a human muscle is cut transversely, the diameter of the **motor unit territory** is roughly 4–12mm, depending on the choice of muscle. During very gentle contraction, when only very few motor units are active, many muscle fibres adjacent to the EMG needle will not fire since they belong to motor units yet to be recruited. This is the best time for the electromyographer to examine the motor unit action potentials generated by muscle fibres from a single motor unit (Box 4.1).

Box 4.1 Basic concepts

Anatomical	**Motor unit:** an anatomical and physiological unit comprising a motor neuron and all the muscle fibres it supplies.
Electrical	**Motor unit action potential:** an electrical signal which is the sum of the potentials generated by those muscle fibres from a single motor unit which are within recording range of the tip of the EMG needle.

The EMG needle records from only a small volume of muscle, yet the motor units recorded cover a large volume, termed the motor unit territory, containing up to several hundred muscle fibres. Some researchers estimate there may be over 1000 muscle fibres in a single motor unit in gastrocnemius. It is clear from this that:

- The needle cannot simultaneously record potentials from all muscle fibres in a motor unit.
- When the needle is moved slightly it will record from different muscle fibres within the same motor unit, so the resulting motor unit action potential will change shape slightly.
- With large needle movement or increased muscle contraction, new motor units altogether are recorded.
- Only a fraction of the muscle is investigated, so occasional false negative results are to be expected in patchy conditions.

A change in the morphology of the motor unit action potential tells us about the configuration of the motor unit, and therefore the type of pathology affecting a muscle. This shall be considered in Chapter 5. First we must understand how a motor unit action potential is measured, what determines its amplitude and duration, and how reliable these measures are.

Measuring a Motor Unit Action Potential

EMG is dynamic, with variation both in needle position and strength of muscle contraction during the examination. With minimal contraction just a few motor units fire, allowing the electromyographer to study the shape of the potentials recorded (Fig. 4.2).

The morphology of the motor unit action potential has multiple determinants. Technical factors include the type of needle and electrical characteristics of the amplifier and filters. Most of these do not need further consideration in this introductory text, but an appreciation of the effect of distance from the needle tip to the muscle fibre is helpful, and is discussed here. Physiological variables include age, choice of muscle, temperature, and strength of contraction, but again they will not be considered further. It is the pathological variables that are, of course, of interest to the clinician, and those of particular interest include:

- Innervation ratio, the number of muscle fibres in the motor unit.
- Fibre density, the number of muscle fibres in a cross-sectional area.
- Muscle fibre diameter and conduction velocity.

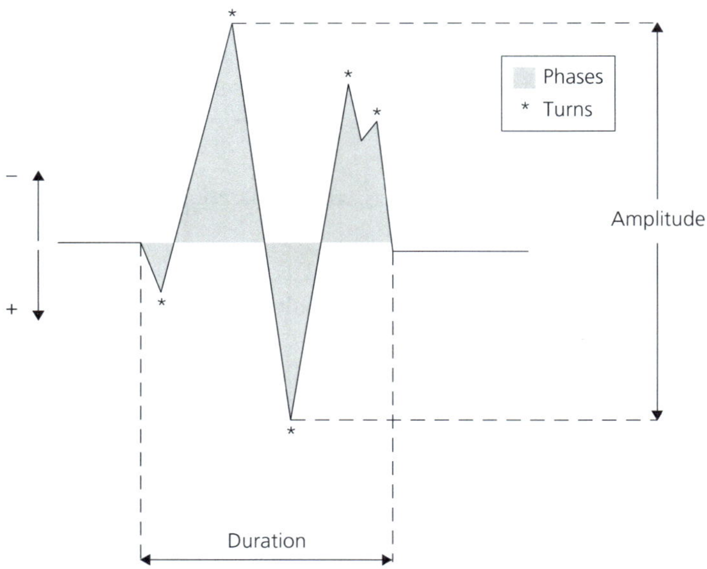

Figure 4.2 The motor unit action potential.

1. Duration: time from the initial deflection away from baseline to the final return to baseline.
2. Amplitude: the maximal peak-to-peak amplitude.
3. Phases: the number of times the potential crosses the baseline plus one.
4. Stability: change in motor unit morphology as it fires repetitively without movement of the EMG needle.

Many of the multiple determinants of motor unit action potential morphology are relatively fixed, allowing us to make some generalizations about the common clinically relevant sources of variation.

Normal range of motor unit action potential morphologies

Amplitude

The amplitude of the motor unit action potential is determined by very few muscle fibres within about 0.5mm of the electrode tip, so it changes with very slight needle movement even though the same motor unit is being recorded (see Table 4.1). Very high amplitude motor unit action potentials are recorded when the needle tip is very close to a dense cluster of synchronously firing muscle fibres (Fig. 4.3).

Table 4.1 Motor unit action potential morphology recorded by concentric needle EMG

	Determinants	Normal value
Amplitude	Synchrony of firing, size and density of muscle fibres at the needle tip Generally determined by <12 muscle fibres within a 0.5mm radius of the concentric needle tip	Commonly 1–4mV, depending on technical factors Varies a lot with needle position
Duration	Number of muscle fibres in a motor unit, and synchrony of firing. It is the parameter that most accurately reflects motor unit territory Determined by muscle fibres within approximately 2mm radius of the needle tip	About 8–12msec, but muscle and age specific Less variation with needle position than amplitude
Phases	Synchrony of muscle fibre action potentials	≤4 But normal muscles may have 10% polyphasic units

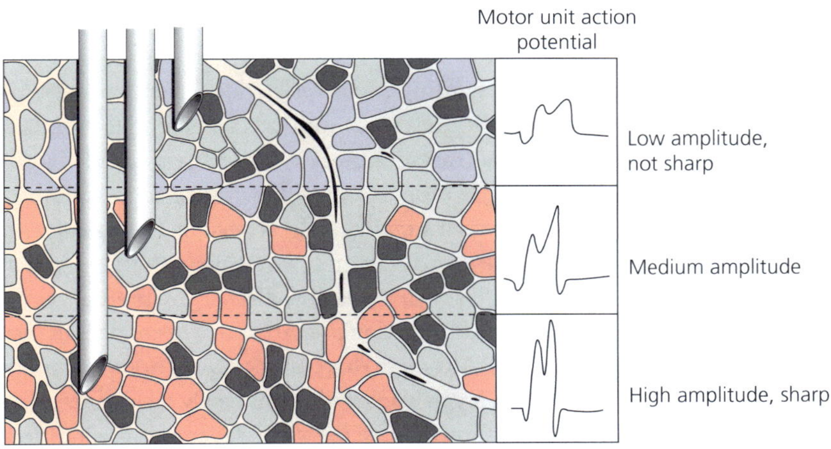

Figure 4.3 EMG needle movement within the motor unit territory affects the shape of the motor unit potential recorded. As the needle gets closer to muscle fibres in the active (red) motor unit, the motor unit action potential becomes higher amplitude.

Duration

Motor unit action potential duration, on the other hand, is determined by a greater number of muscle fibres, from a radius of up to 2mm from the electrode tip. It is therefore rather less affected by slight changes in needle position than amplitude. Duration of the motor unit action potential is abnormal in neurogenic and myopathic conditions (Chapter 5), and is the most reliable correlate of motor unit territory. Increased motor unit action potential duration can occur as a result of an increase in the total number of muscle fibres in a motor unit, or desynchronization of existing muscle fibre action potentials. Decreased duration occurs due to loss of a proportion of muscle fibres from a motor unit, which may be anatomical or physiological (due to terminal conduction block causing a proportion of fibres to be inactive).

Phases

Polyphasic motor unit action potentials arise because of a loss of synchrony of firing of the muscle fibres close to the tip of the recording needle. They are seen in both neurogenic and myopathic conditions, discussed in Chapter 5. Usually only a small proportion of the motor unit action potentials recorded from a muscle are polyphasic (up to about 10%). Occasionally, particularly when there is reinnervation, small potentials are seen which are time locked to the main motor unit action potential, termed '**satellite potentials**'. The delay in their activation commonly reflects a long distal nerve terminal, and a narrow diameter or immature distal nerve.

Stability

In normal individuals if the recording needle electrode is kept entirely still there is no appreciable variability in motor unit action potential morphology with successive activations (the variability is sometimes called '**jiggle**', which is distinct from '**jitter**'). In other words, following an action potential in a motor axon, the muscle fibres it supplies are activated in a fixed sequence relative to each other with successive discharges. Variation in the morphology of the motor unit action potential with successive discharges implies there is variation in the timing of muscle fibre action potentials due to changes in neuromuscular transmission times. Although this commonly occurs with disease of the neuromuscular junction it can also result from newly formed terminal nerve branches, such as with those associated with denervating conditions where there is remodelling of surviving motor units.

Introducing EMG During Normal Muscle Contraction

To understand the EMG appearances in disease it is necessary first to understand the normal EMG examination, and to introduce the concepts of spontaneous electrical activity, motor unit **recruitment**, and interference pattern, to be expanded on in Chapter 5. To reach a correct conclusion about EMG findings the electromyographer must assimilate the information from a number of different aspects of the examination. Key aspects are highlighted in the following text, but this list is not exhaustive.

Muscle fibres are usually electrically silent at rest. A brief burst of insertional activity is seen when the EMG needle is inserted into the muscle, followed by silence because there is no **spontaneous activity.** In healthy muscle the only exception to this is if the needle happens to lie close to the neuromuscular junction, in which case there may be normal spontaneous **end-plate activity** associated with pain.

With gentle muscle contraction the first motor units to fire are small, usually consisting of relatively thin motor axons contacting a small number of type I muscle fibres. In limb muscles, the initial firing rate of these motor units is approximately 5–8Hz. It is during weak contraction that the electromyographer moves the needle to assess the **morphology of different motor unit action potentials**.

To generate a more forceful contraction, the firing rate of the first recorded motor unit increases until, at about 7–10 Hz for limb muscles, higher for facial muscles, another unit is recruited which initially fires slowly. With increasing force of contraction the motor units already firing do so at higher rates, fastest in those motor units recruited earliest, and slower for larger motor units recruited late. The force of contraction is therefore increased both by increasing the firing **frequency** of active units, and by orderly recruitment of successively larger and stronger motor units. Assessment of this **recruitment pattern** is an essential part of the EMG examination, and is altered by pathology that affects the size or number of motor units that can be activated, or by a change in the central drive to the alpha motor neurons.

The last motor units recruited are the biggest, many of which will have large-diameter axons innervating type II muscle fibres. On EMG these correspond to higher-amplitude, longer-duration motor unit action potentials than those initially recruited. In normal muscle these large motor units are difficult to examine since they are recruited last, into an already busy EMG screen. It is for this reason that EMG is relatively insensitive to pathology that predominantly affects type II muscle fibres if type I fibres are spared. Usually the EMG screen shows a full **interference pattern** when a normal muscle is contracted strongly.

Chapter 5

Deconstructing the EMG: Origin of Abnormalities

Key points

- No single EMG abnormality is specific for a particular pathology.
- Spontaneous EMG activity, recorded from a resting muscle, originates from the motor nerve, neuromuscular junction, or muscle fibre.
- The origin and type of spontaneous EMG activity may be identified by studying the firing pattern and morphology of the waveform.
- Normal end-plate activity is important to identify and exclude: it disappears with slight needle movement, as does the pain experienced by the patient.
- Myopathies are characterized by small motor units due to the loss of muscle fibres. The result is short-duration, low-amplitude, polyphasic motor unit action potentials.
- Partial axon loss results in remodelling of surviving motor units, which become abnormally large. Needle EMG reveals long-duration, high-amplitude, polyphasic motor unit action potentials.
- With muscle contraction the recruitment of motor units is 'reduced' in neurogenic lesions—a smaller number of motor units fire than expected, and they do so at high rates in relative isolation.
- In myopathies recruitment of the abnormally small motor unit action potentials is 'early' or 'rapid'—a greater number of motor units are active than expected for the force of contraction since individually they are so weak.
- Motor unit action potential morphology is normal in muscles that are weak due to upper motor neuron lesions or conduction block of peripheral motor nerves. However, there are abnormalities of motor unit recruitment.

EMG is a dynamic procedure, best appreciated in real time whilst feeling the force generated by the muscle under examination. The electromyographer concentrates on four key aspects of the EMG signal: spontaneous activity with the muscle relaxed, the morphology of motor unit action potentials, their recruitment as the muscle is activated, and finally, the interference pattern with strong contraction.

This chapter takes a deconstructive approach to the EMG, breaking it down to enable an understanding of the range of abnormalities seen in each of these four parameters in turn. Understanding the anatomical and physiological bases of these abnormalities enables us to interpret both typical and unexpected findings, and predict the underlying pathology. Although referring clinicians who may never perform EMG do not need to remember the detail of this chapter, an understanding of the basic principles helps with the interpretation of tricky cases.

Since no single EMG finding is specific for a disease or type of pathology the electromyographer recognizes patterns of abnormality in order to determine pathology. This constructive approach is taken in Chapter 6, which will also highlight some of the pitfalls to interpreting EMG parameters in isolation.

Spontaneous Activity

A normal muscle should be electrically silent at rest unless the needle is at the end plate. Spontaneous activity refers to electrical discharges recorded with the patient completely relaxed in the absence of EMG needle movement. The electromyographer must be able to determine the type of spontaneous activity, and from where it is generated; identify normal end-plate activity; and understand the clinical associations with different types of spontaneous activity.

Origin and types of spontaneous activity

Spontaneous activity is generated at one of three sites: the peripheral nerve, neuromuscular junction, or the muscle fibre itself. It is usually relatively straightforward to tell them apart by learning to recognize the characteristic sounds and by studying:

- Duration and complexity (primarily number of phases) of the potential.
- Firing rate and pattern.
- Direction of the initial deflection of the potential from baseline.

Single muscle fibre discharges are very brief in duration, less than 5ms, and are simple in morphology, usually biphasic (see Table 5.1). Usually the initial deflection is positive (downwards) since the action potential travels towards, then away from, the needle. However, if the needle is right at the end plate the **muscle fibre action potential** is initiated directly beneath the needle, with the result that the brief positive deflection may be absent and therefore the initial deflection may be negative (upwards). Single fibre potentials are briefer and generally of lower amplitude than the combined potentials recorded from a motor unit—the motor unit action potential.

Fibrillation potentials are one of the most important EMG findings. They arise due to denervation of single muscle fibres and can occur in neurogenic or myopathic conditions, and occasionally even with neuromuscular junction pathology. They arise due to reorganization of acetylcholine receptors following denervation, resulting in hypersensitivity. Over time the tendency to fibrillate reduces, but fibrillation potentials can be seen in longstanding disease, for example, they are sometimes seen many years after poliomyelitis. It therefore may be misguiding to report **fibrillations** as evidence of 'acute denervation', although they presumably do reflect some degree of ongoing disease activity or motor unit remodelling even though it may be minimal. When fibrillation potentials and/or **positive sharp waves** are encountered it is common practice to grade how profuse they are:

0: none.
+1: single trains of potentials in at least two areas.
+2: moderate numbers of potentials in at least three areas.
+3: many potentials in all areas.
+4: full interference pattern of potentials.

Peripheral nerve discharges, arising anywhere from the cell body to distal axon, will cause activation of the whole motor unit (see Table 5.2). The resultant motor unit action potential recorded on EMG is of longer duration than a single muscle fibre discharge, usually about 10–12ms, since it represents the sum of several muscle fibre potentials. It tends to be of greater amplitude and have more phases than a single muscle fibre potential.

Neuromuscular junction activity is only recorded at the end plate, and is low amplitude and easily missed unless the amplification is increased (see Table 5.3). The tiny rounded potentials (<40uV) represent spontaneous release of vesicles of acetylcholine which cause **miniature end-plate potentials** insufficient to reach threshold and trigger a muscle fibre action potential.

Table 5.1 Spontaneous EMG activity originating from single muscle fibres

Origin	Discharge type	Morphology	Firing rate and pattern	Associations
Single muscle fibre	End-plate spike (normal)	1. The initial deflection is often –ve implying the action potential originates under the needle tip 2. Usually biphasic, <5ms <200μV 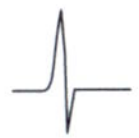	*Irregular* firing rate, often high frequency 5–50Hz 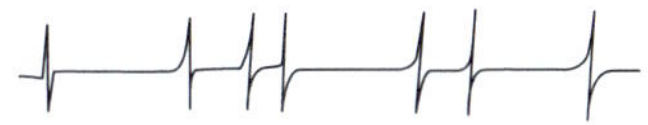	Normal, caused by mechanical activation of the nerve terminal—painful
(Increasing instability ... *continued*)	Positive sharp wave	Initial short +ve deflection with following longer low-amplitude negative component. Often up to 10–30ms duration 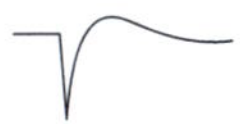	*Regular* firing—helps to differentiate from end-plate spikes. 0.5–10Hz 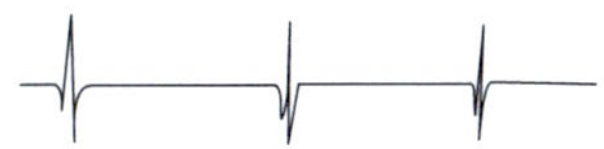	Any cause of denervation of a muscle fibre: *Neuropathic (common):* anterior horn cell disease, radiculopathy, axonal neuropathy, nerve transection *Myopathic*: especially inflammatory myopathies, dystrophies, some toxic, metabolic and congenital myopathies. *Neuromuscular junction (less common)*: botulism, severe myasthenia, or Lambert–Eaton myasthenic syndrome
	Fibrillation potential	Initial +ve deflection often, suggesting that the needle is not at the end plate. <5ms duration. 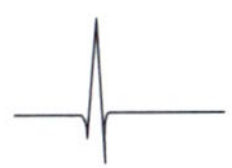		

(Continued)

Table 5.1 (Continued)

Origin	Discharge type	Morphology	Firing rate and pattern	Associations
↓	Myotonia	Individual potentials look either like positive sharp waves or fibrillation potentials. Increased if the muscle is tapped or the needle moved slightly	Wax and wane ('divebomber sound') 40–100Hz 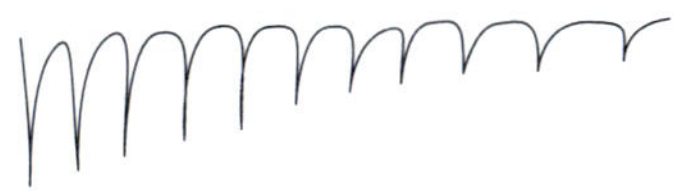	*With clinical myotonia*: myotonic dystrophy 1 & 2, myotonia congenita, paramyotonia congenita *No clinical myotonia*: hyperkalaemic periodic paralysis, polymyositis, acid maltase deficiency, toxic. *Neurogenic*: rare in severe axonal disorders.
Several muscle fibres	Complex repetitive discharge	An abnormal local circuit within the muscle activating adjacent single fibres. Thus each discharge looks like a cluster of grouped fibrillation potentials of different sizes 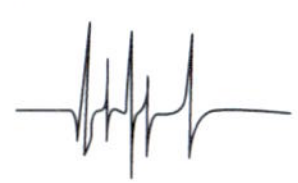	Each polyphasic discharge is identical to the last (same excitatory circuit). Regular firing frequency, sudden onset & offset. Machinery sound. 3–40Hz 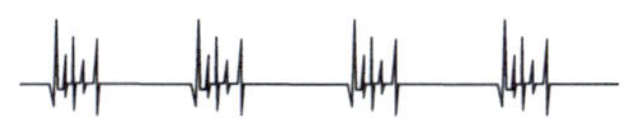	Occurs when there is adjacent muscle fibre denervation. *Chronic neurogenic*: radiculopathies, neuropathies, anterior horn cell disease *Chronic myopathies*: inflammatory, muscular dystrophy. Rarely in normal biceps, iliopsoas

Table 5.2 Spontaneous EMG activity originating from motor axons

Origin	Discharge type	Morphology	Firing rate and pattern	Associations
Motor axon (so whole motor unit activated)	Fasciculation potential	Often initial positive deflection. Broader and taller than a fibrillation potential since all fibres of a motor unit are activated (spontaneous equivalent of the motor unit action potential) 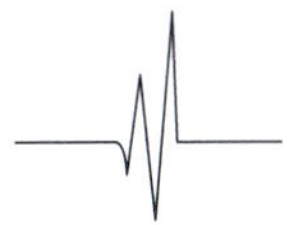	Slow and *irregular*, usually <2Hz (thus not confused with voluntary activity—rare to activate units voluntarily at <4Hz) 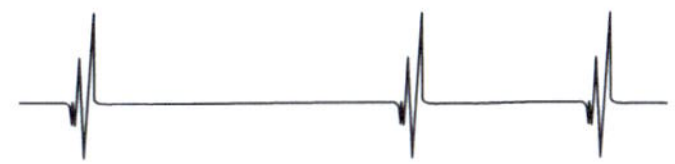	Majority thought to originate from distal axon rather than cell body Common with 'neurogenic pathology' anywhere from cell body to distal axon. Also cramp fasciculation syndrome, hyperthyroidism, anticholinesterase drugs Can be normal, so not significant if seen in isolation
(Increasing instability)	Doublets and triplets	Individual units the same morphology as fasciculations, but occurring in pairs, triplets or multiplets.	1–50Hz usually intraburst 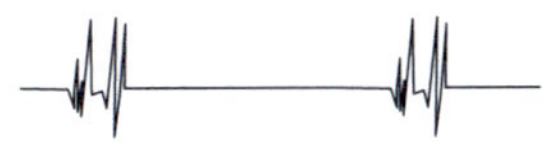	
	Myokymia	Individual units the same morphology as fasciculations. Thought to represent spontaneous depolarization along demyelinated segments of nerve	Bursts of firing with sudden onset/offset and no waxing or waning. Sounds like 'marching soldiers'. <10Hz interburst 40–60Hz intraburst 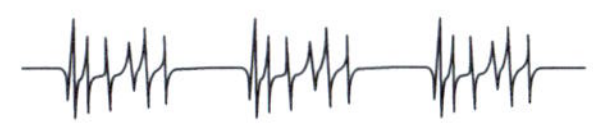	*Limbs*: radiation injury, chronic nerve entrapment, chronic radiculopathy, Isaac's syndrome, Morvan's syndrome. *Facial muscles*: AIDP, multiple sclerosis, pontine glioma, CIDP. Not always associated with clinical myokymia

(Continued)

Table 5.2 (Continued)

Origin	Discharge type	Morphology	Firing rate and pattern	Associations
↓	Neuromyotonia	Individual units the same morphology as fasciculations if discharges are slowed and examined in detail	100–300Hz Decrementing, makes a 'pinging' sound (not affected by muscle activity) 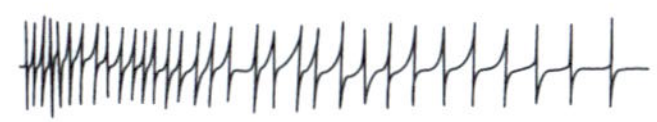	Often accompanied by fasciculations and myokymia. Isaac's syndrome, Morvan's syndrome, hyperhydrosis. Also very chronic neuropathies, adult SMA, old polio.
Several motor units	Cramp	Motor units look essentially normal	Rapid build-up of full interference pattern, spluttering offset 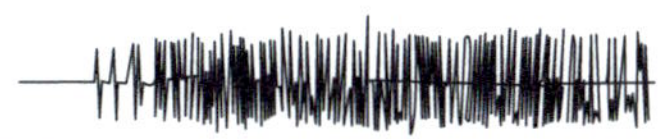	Triggered by contraction of a muscle that is already in its shortened position. Origin is axon not muscle

AIDP, acute inflammatory demyelinating polyneuropathy; CIDP, chronic inflammatory demyelinating polyneuropathy.

Table 5.3 Spontaneous EMG activity originating from the neuromuscular junction

Origin	Discharge type	Morphology	Firing rate and pattern	Associations
Neuromuscular junction	Miniature end-plate potential (end-plate noise)	Tiny rounded fluctuations of the baseline, up to 40uV, <2ms duration 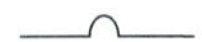	Continuous irregular firing ('white noise' sound—like a seashell) 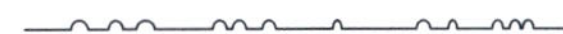	Normal —the needle at the end plate causes pain

Normal end-plate activity

It is important that end-plate activity is recognized since it is normal. In clinical practice this is usually straightforward since there are two clues: the patient complains of more pain than usual, and with slight needle movement both the pain and the spontaneous activity disappear.

End-plate activity takes one of two forms. Spontaneous release of quanta of acetylcholine causes **end-plate noise** which sounds like the faint hiss on listening to a sea shell. Single muscle fibre discharges, on the other hand, cause end-plate spikes that superficially look rather like fibrillation potentials, but can usually be distinguished by their initial negative (upwards) deflection and their fast irregular firing rate.

Motor Unit Action Potential Morphology

The motor unit action potential is determined by several muscle fibre action potentials from a single motor unit, but does not reflect activity of all the muscle fibres in that motor unit (see Chapter 4). At its most basic level the motor unit (not the motor unit action potential, which is the electrical measurement as opposed to the anatomical structure) can either be abnormally small, in which case an action potential activates fewer muscle fibres than expected, or abnormally large, where very many muscle fibres are activated by a single axon.

Small motor units in myopathies

Abnormally small motor units tend to be found in myopathies, where muscle pathology results in loss or dysfunction of a proportion of muscle fibres (see Table 5.4). In a myopathy, motor unit action potential duration is short because of a reduction in the number of muscle fibres in the motor unit, with little change in the synchrony of their firing. Amplitude is reduced since there is less constructive interference given there is a reduction in the number of muscle fibre action potentials. The muscle fibres themselves may also be thinner diameter than normal and may be present at a lower density at the needle tip than in normal muscle, contributing to the loss of amplitude. The loss of many muscle fibres means that the low-amplitude, short-duration motor unit action potential may also be polyphasic.

It is important to appreciate that any reason for a loss of transmission of a proportion of the terminal axon branches to individual muscle fibres, or some of the neuromuscular junctions, can cause functional loss of a number of muscle fibres and thus cause 'myopathic-looking' motor unit action potentials. An example is the motor unit action potentials seen in severe myasthenia or botulism, but similar morphologies may be seen with early 'nascent'

Table 5.4 Origin of normal and abnormal motor unit action potential morphology (see Chapter 6 for a summary of EMG findings with pathology)

		Normal	Myopathic	Neuropathic
Pathology ○ = Normal muscle fibre ◌ = Degenerated ○ = Reinnervated		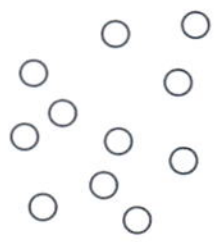	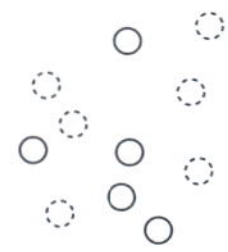	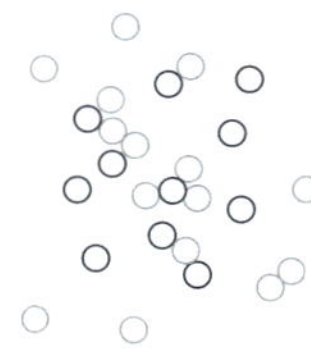
Electrical	Single muscle fibre potentials	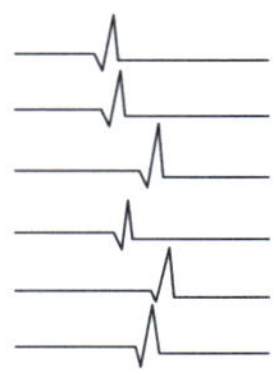	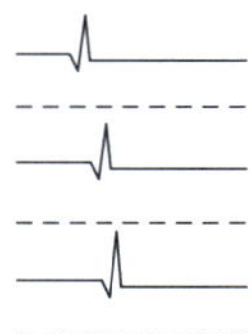	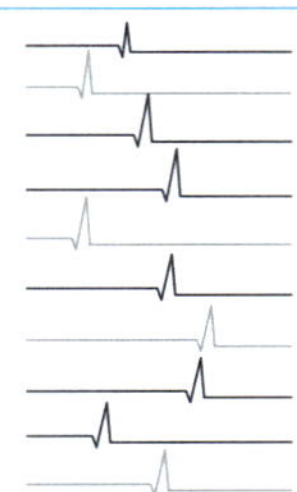
	MUAP	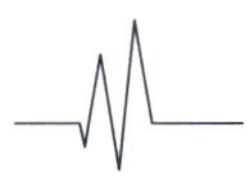	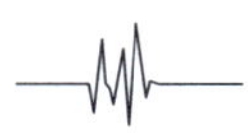	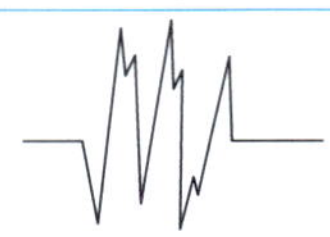
	Duration	Normal	Short	Long
	Amplitude	Normal	Low	High
	Phases	Normal	Often ↑	Often ↑
Other causes of similar MUAP morphology		Normal	Also seen with reinnervation ('nascent units') and partial NMJ blockade.	Also seen in some chronic myopathies e.g. inclusion body myositis

MUAP: Motor unit action potential; NMJ: neuromuscular junction.

regenerating motor units after **axonotmesis** (although these often also have late 'satellite potentials'). Usually of course the clinical presentations distinguish these possibilities, but EMG differences in spontaneous activity, stability, and recruitment pattern will also be seen, discussed in Chapter 6.

Large motor units with neurogenic pathology

Large motor units are generated by sprouting of terminal axons to innervate nearby muscle fibres which have lost their usual nerve supply. This can result in unusually dense clusters of muscle fibres sharing a common innervation, and thus firing relatively synchronously. When these are close to the needle tip the result is an abnormally high amplitude motor unit action potential.

The number of muscle fibres in the motor unit is increased, as is its territory, reflected in an increase in the duration of the motor unit action potential. The new axons and immature neuromuscular junctions are often slower, and initially rather less reliable, than long-established neuromuscular connections, contributing to the polyphasia, long duration, and instability of the motor unit action potential.

Although large motor units are characteristically seen in longstanding neurogenic disease following loss of a proportion of motor axons, they can also be seen in chronic myopathies where there has been intramuscular damage to terminal motor axons, or muscle fibre splitting and subsequent remodelling of motor units. It is common for long-duration motor unit action potentials to have high amplitude, but this is not inevitable, and therefore to talk of 'large' versus 'small' potentials is less accurate than describing both their amplitude and duration.

Recruitment Pattern

Recruitment can be defined as 'the successive activation of the same and additional motor units with increasing strength of voluntary muscle contraction'(1). There are only two ways to increase the force of muscular contraction:

1. The firing frequency of muscle fibres can be increased.
2. More muscle fibres can be activated.

Muscle fibres are organized structurally and functionally into motor units, which vary in size in normal muscle, but even more so in disease. Small motor units, with few muscle fibres, provide a weaker contractile force than large motor units. It makes sense, therefore, to activate the smallest motor units first in healthy muscle, thereby generating a low force for fine precision movement. As the required force of muscle contraction increases, successively larger motor units become active according to Henneman's size principle, whilst the firing frequency of already active units increases.

When the electromyographer examines recruitment pattern they do so as the force of contraction is slowly increased. Initially they concentrate on the motor units activated first with minimal contraction, and whether they are the relatively small motor units expected. Next, as the contraction is increased very slightly, attention is paid to how rapidly the existing motor units fire as another is recruited. As the muscle becomes more strongly contracted the electromyographer notes how many motor units are firing, and at what frequency, in relation to that expected in a normal muscle given the force of contraction.

Normal recruitment

- *Size*. In normal muscles small motor units are activated first, with large motor units only becoming active during strong contraction. Hence the EMG is relatively insensitive to isolated type II muscle fibre pathology since these fibres generally occur in large motor units and are only activated once there is a relatively full interference pattern.
- *Rate*. The first motor unit usually initially fires at 4–8Hz, although some irregular firing as slow as 2–3Hz is occasionally seen. Once it fires at about 8–10Hz (higher for facial muscles), a second is recruited which initially fires at about 5Hz. Once the first unit gets to about 15Hz there are usually three or more units firing, and so on (the 'rule of fives'). A motor unit usually increases firing rate to 20–40Hz as patient effort increases.

Recruitment can only occur in the expected orderly fashion provided there is:

- Normal *central drive* via the brain and spinal cord to determine firing rate and recruitment of anterior horn cells. This can be affected by pain, lack of volition, and upper motor neuron lesions.
- A normal complement of *motor units*, some small which will activate early, and some larger and only recruited during forceful contraction (generally larger axons innervating type II muscle fibres).

Abnormal recruitment

As with other abnormalities of the EMG signal, it is important to appreciate that no recruitment pattern is specific to a single pathology. For example, rapid recruitment may be seen whenever there are many small motor units, and is most commonly observed in myopathies. However, it can also be seen in severe neuromuscular junction disease where the motor units are rendered functionally small due to failure of transmission at some junctions. Likewise, reduced recruitment, most commonly associated with a reduced motor unit pool due to axonal pathology, may be observed in a chronic myopathy if entire motor units are lost and the survivors are large, such as can occur in muscular dystrophies.

Abnormal motor units, normal central drive

Reduced recruitment in neurogenic lesions Following degeneration of a proportion of anterior horn cells or their axons, there are fewer motor units than normal, and those that remain are larger than normal because of remodelling. During relatively gentle contraction surprisingly large motor units are recruited early because of the lack of normal smaller units. As the force of contraction is increased the firing rate of the unit already active is higher than normal before a second unit is recruited, called a high '**recruitment frequency**' (see Table 5.5).

There comes a point when no more motor units are available to be recruited, so the electromyographer sees relatively few motor unit action potentials (which are long duration, high amplitude and polyphasic) firing at high rates in relative isolation—'reduced recruitment'. Compare this to the recruitment pattern when there is peripheral motor conduction block.

Early, or rapid, recruitment in myopathy

Myopathies cause a reduction in the size, and therefore strength, of motor units, so it makes sense that to compensate for this more will need to be active. So when the electromyographer examines a weakly contracting myopathic muscle more motor unit action potentials are seen than normal (and they are short duration, low amplitude and polyphasic). In this situation the recruitment frequency is relatively normal (the rate at which an active unit fires before another is activated). '**Early recruitment**' (also termed 'rapid recruitment') refers to the greater number of motor units active than expected for the force of contraction of that muscle.

As the patient tries to increase the force of contraction, all available motor units fire even though the muscle is still weakly contracting.

Abnormal recruitment despite normal motor units

Poor activation due to reduced central drive If there is a lack of central drive to the anterior horn cells for any reason, for example, pain, lack of volition, or an upper motor neuron lesion, the recruitment pattern is normal initially. Small motor units are recruited first, followed by slightly larger ones in an orderly fashion. However, at the point that central drive plateaus there will be no further recruitment of motor units *and* there will be no increase in the firing rate of those already recruited: the recruitment pattern is described as 'poor activation' (see Table 5.6).

Thus, although recruitment frequency and pattern are initially normal, there are relatively few units firing, although they do so at rates appropriate for the force of contraction. Contrast this with recruitment in a weak muscle due to a neurogenic lesion, in which few motor units fire fast (furthermore, their morphology is abnormal). EMG alone cannot distinguish the cause for a lack of central drive, but of course there are generally other clinical clues.

Peripheral conduction block with intact central drive

When there is partial motor conduction block affecting the peripheral nerve, the initial motor units activated may appear normal, or nearly so, depending

Table 5.5 Recruitment pattern with abnormal motor units, normal central drive

	Normal	**Neurogenic**	**Myopathic**
Number of motor units	N	↓	N
Size of motor units	N	↑	↓
Central drive	N	N	N
Recruitment	*Normal*: orderly activation of progressively larger motor units to a full interference pattern with strong contraction	*Reduced*: with maximal effort only few motor units fire, but they do so at high rates (in a weak muscle)	*Rapid/early*: with weak contraction many more motor units are active than normal since they are individually weak (as is muscle strength)
Weak contraction → Strong contraction	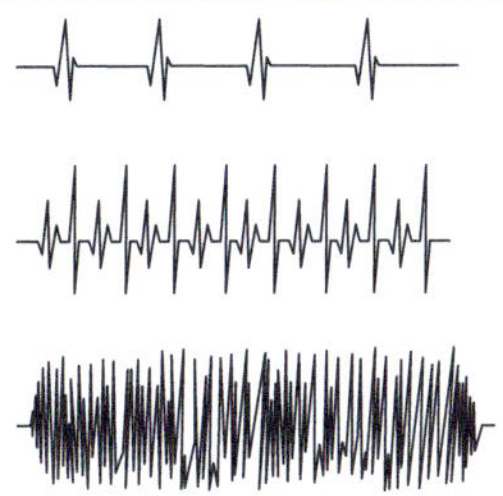	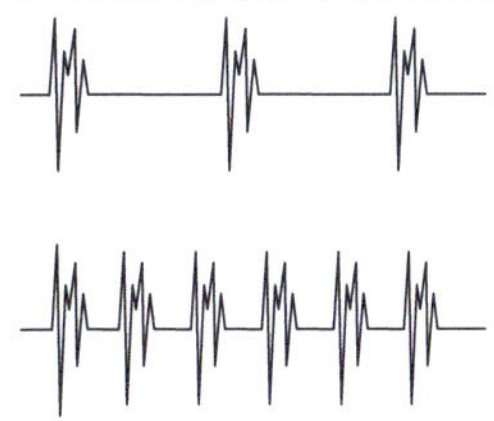	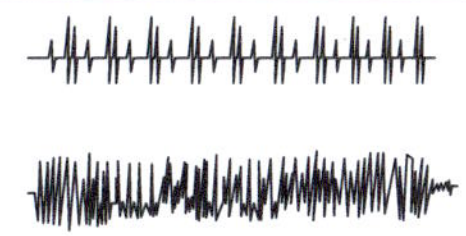
Interference pattern	N	↓	Full, but low amplitude

N, normal; ↓, decreased; ↑, increased.

Table 5.6 Recruitment pattern with abnormal central drive, normal motor units

	Normal	**Upper motor neuron lesion, pain, volitional**	**Peripheral conduction block**
Number of motor units	N	N	N, but only a fraction can be activated
Size of motor units	N	N	N
Central drive	N	↓	N
Recruitment	*Normal*: orderly activation of progressively larger motor units to a full interference pattern with strong contraction	*Poor activation*: recruitment is initially normal, but full activation is not achieved. Firing rate is normal for the number of motor units active and the low force of contraction	*Reduced*: with maximal effort only few motor units fire, but they do so at high rates (in a weak muscle)
Weak contraction → Strong contraction	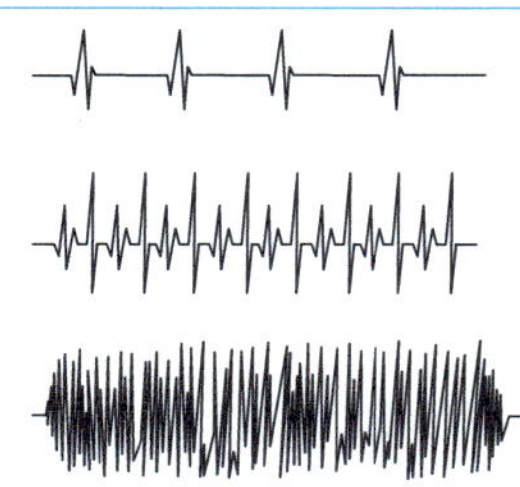	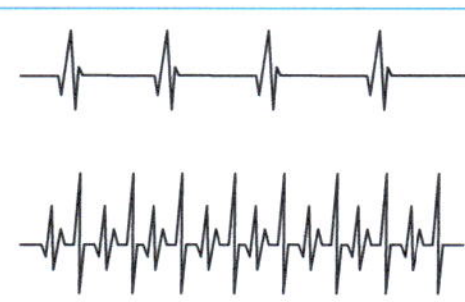	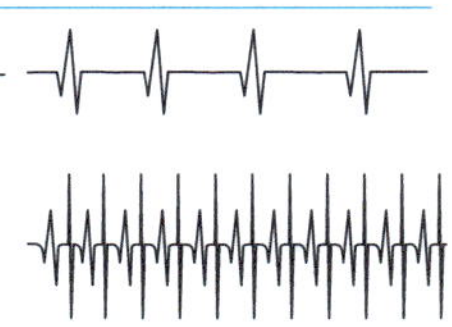
Interference pattern	N	↓	↓

N, normal; ↓, decreased.

on which units, and how many, are blocked. As the force of contraction is increased there comes a point at which all available motor units are active. As force of contraction increases beyond this there is no problem with central drive, so with maximal exertion the available motor units fire very rapidly in relative isolation—and of course the muscle remains weak.

Just like with neurogenic pathology there is reduced recruitment, with fewer motor units than normal firing at high rates in relative isolation. The rate of firing will be disproportionately high compared to the number of motor units firing, and there is a reduction in the total number of motor units recruited.

It may be distinguished from the neurogenic EMG since morphology of the motor unit action potentials is normal with pure conduction block, and there are no fibrillation potentials. In reality, secondary axonal loss may complicate the picture.

Interference Pattern

Once recruitment is understood, the EMG interference pattern in different conditions follows logically since it is the result of maximal exertion. Achieving a full interference pattern requires both adequate central drive and a normal number of motor units. When recording interference pattern the electromyographer pays particular attention to:

- The degree of obliteration of the baseline of the record, and
- The amplitude of the interference pattern. This is rather less susceptible to needle movement than the amplitude of single motor unit action potentials since it is determined by many such potentials.

In a neurogenic lesion the interference pattern is reduced, with abnormally high amplitude, polyphasic, long-duration motor unit action potentials firing at high rates but with appreciable brief gaps in between them. This gives a very characteristic juddering sound.

In contrast, with myopathic pathology there is a full interference pattern despite a weak contraction, and although the individual motor unit action potentials cannot be discerned, the amplitude of the interference pattern is lower than normal.

Patients with peripheral motor conduction block or a lack of central drive will have a reduced interference pattern but they may be told apart by the recruitment and firing patterns already discussed, and of course their different clinical presentation.

Reference

1. AAEM glossary of terms in electrodiagnostic medicine. *Muscle Nerve 2001*, **24**(Supplement 10), s5–s28.

Chapter 6

Axis 1: Pathology

Key points

- Nerve conduction and EMG must be reviewed together— patterns of abnormality reveal the type of pathology, isolated findings are not specific and must be interpreted in context.
- In general, nerve conduction and EMG examine the more resilient surviving axons and muscle fibres, not necessarily those most affected by disease.
- Nerve conduction response amplitude, conduction velocity, and degree of temporal dispersion allow assessment of axon loss versus demyelination. This may be confirmed with EMG.
- Demyelination generally results in conduction slowing. There is relative preservation of response amplitude unless there is conduction block, temporal dispersion, or secondary axon loss.
- Marked conduction slowing (<70% of normal) implies demyelination even if the CMAP is small. EMG can help detect additional axon loss.
- There are many causes of a low-amplitude CMAP—it does not imply axonal pathology and should be interpreted with other neurophysiological findings, particularly EMG.
- Fibrillation potentials are not specific for acute denervation. For example, they may be present in chronic neurogenic disease, and in some myopathies.
- Long-duration, high-amplitude, polyphasic motor unit action potentials are typical of neurogenic conditions but may be seen in myopathies. Small, polyphasic potentials are typical of myopathies, but can be seen with reinnervation after axonal loss. The key to making the correct diagnosis is the wider context, electrophysiological and clinical.

The diseases commonly seen in the neurophysiological laboratory can be divided along the length of the neuraxis into those that affect upper motor neurons, lower motor neurons, the neuromuscular junction, and muscle. Disease of each of these components can be distinguished by patterns of change in nerve conduction and EMG—in many ways similar to localization in the clinical neurology examination according to patterns of weakness and reflex changes. The purpose of this chapter is to provide an overview of how patterns of abnormalities in nerve conduction (Chapter 3) and EMG (Chapter 5) may be interpreted together to determine what type of pathology is present. The aim is therefore to emphasize abnormal patterns that must be recognized. Readers unfamiliar with nerve conduction and EMG should review the earlier chapters before returning.

No single change in nerve conduction or EMG parameters is specific for a particular pathology; rather it is the pattern of abnormalities that matters. For example, although spontaneous fibrillation potentials are commonly found with needle EMG after acute axonal lesions, they can also be seen in some myopathies, in which case the wider EMG context is different and they will be accompanied by small polyphasic motor unit action potentials that recruit rapidly with weak contraction. Without knowing the wider neurophysiological and clinical context it is easy to misinterpret findings.

With experience, the electrophysiologist rapidly becomes familiar with predicting and spotting the patterns considered in this chapter. Since it is often straightforward to determine which section of the neuraxis is diseased, the objective of the examining neurophysiologist then shifts towards gauging the severity of that pathology, detecting subclinical lesions, and showing the extent of disease. Since the localization of disease often requires particular effort, and commonly determines the duration and extent of the examination, it will be considered separately in Chapter 7.

Nerve Conduction Studies: Interpret with EMG

Remember the basic rule that *axonal pathology results in a loss of response amplitude, whereas demyelination causes conduction slowing* (see Chapter 3 for further details). To interpret nerve conduction results correctly it is important to know the amplitude of responses, degree of temporal dispersion, and the conduction velocities along the length of the nerve. This allows a judgement to be made about the relative contributions of axon loss and demyelination, since it is not uncommon for pathology to be mixed. This is then generally confirmed with EMG. Table 6.1 provides a summary of the patterns of abnormality expected with different pathologies. Nerve conduction is particularly

Table 6.1 Nerve conduction and EMG with peripheral nerve pathology

		Axon loss	Focal demyelination		Diffuse homogeneous demyelination
			Conduction block	Temporal dispersion	
Sensory (SNAP)	Amplitude	↓↓	N when stimulation and recording sites are both distal to the lesion		N, or ↓ due to temporal dispersion
	Conduction velocity	N*	N (as above)		↓↓↓
Motor (CMAP)	Amplitude	↓↓	↓ amplitude and area when stimulation is proximal to the lesion and recording distal. No temporal dispersion	Temporal dispersion, so ↓ amplitude but area unchanged with stimulation proximal to the lesion and recording distal	N, or ↓ slightly due to temporal dispersion and secondary axonal loss
	Conduction velocity	N*	↓ across the lesion usually	↓ commonly	↓↓↓
EMG		Broad, tall, polyphasic motor unit action potentials, reduced recruitment	Normal motor unit action potentials, reduced recruitment	Relatively normal	Relatively normal, unless secondary axonal loss

N, normal; * with severe axonal pathology, the loss of fast large-diameter fibres can result in mild slowing of conduction velocity; ↓, decreased; ↓↓, moderately decreased, ↓↓↓, severely decreased; SNAP, sensory nerve action potential; CMAP, compound muscle action potential.

helpful for conditions affecting the nerves between their spinal root and the neuromuscular junction, but is less instructive when pathology is either very proximal or distal.

There are, of course, exceptions, or at least qualifications, to the basic rules. Demyelination may result in a reduction of the sensory or motor response amplitude in a number of settings:

- Patchy demyelination may cause desynchronization of individual action potentials, termed 'temporal dispersion'. The response duration is prolonged and amplitude reduced, but the area remains relatively unchanged.

- Focal demyelination/dysfunction at the nodes of Ranvier may result in conduction block, in which case the response amplitude is significantly smaller when stimulating on the opposite side of the lesion to the recording electrodes.
- With chronic demyelination there is often secondary axon loss, and the resulting denervation will be detected on EMG.

In the context of a demyelinating neuropathy with low response amplitudes, EMG may be helpful in determining whether there is secondary axon loss, or whether the loss of CMAP amplitude simply reflects desynchronization or conduction block. EMG evidence of denervation confirms axon loss, which is clinically important since it is an important determinant of disability and may imply a slower recovery. Thus it is the overall pattern of nerve conduction and EMG findings that helps determine the relative contribution of demyelination and axon loss.

Sometimes the reverse problem is encountered—there is conduction slowing in a predominantly axonal neuropathy. Axonal pathology causes a loss of sensory or motor response amplitude, but conduction velocity may be marginally reduced in severe disease since there is loss of the fastest conducting fibres. When interpreting a mixed picture, with evidence of both loss of response amplitude and conduction slowing, it is helpful to first consider whether any of the conduction velocities are sufficiently slow to provide definite evidence of demyelination. If there is slowing below 70% of the lower limit of normal this is generally accepted as convincing evidence of demyelination even with small response amplitudes. If sensory or motor response amplitudes remain nearly normal, implying little if any axon loss, a lesser degree of slowing, perhaps to 80–90% of the lower limit of normal, may be sufficient to confidently diagnose demyelination.

EMG: Recognizing Patterns to Determine Pathology

This section consolidates knowledge from Chapter 5, and reinforces how an EMG diagnosis is derived from recognition of patterns of spontaneous activity, motor unit action potential morphology, recruitment, and interference patterns. No single EMG abnormality is specific for a disease, so the EMG must be considered as a whole, and in the context of the nerve conduction results, in order to reach a conclusion about the underlying pathology. Of course a final clinical diagnosis can only be made once the three axes of the neurophysiological examination, that is, the type of pathology, its localization, and time course, are considered in light of the clinical presentation (see Chapters 6–8).

Neurogenic EMG

'Neurogenic change' is seen on EMG following a lesion of the motor nerve anywhere along its length, or due to degeneration of the anterior horn cell body itself (see Table 6.2). By determining the distribution of axon loss the electromyographer is able to help diagnose numerous conditions including motor neuron disease, radiculopathies, and axonal neuropathies. This brief section considers neurogenic change several weeks after axonal injury, but the evolution of EMG changes with **Wallerian degeneration**, and subsequent nerve regeneration, is important enough to warrant a separate section, and is discussed in Chapter 8.

The EMG findings described here are most commonly seen as a result of primary axonal pathology, but it is important to look at the wider clinical and neurophysiological context. Broad, high-amplitude, polyphasic motor unit action potentials are sometimes seen in myopathic conditions as discussed later. The wider pattern of EMG appearances usually provides a clue to the myopathic pathology: some small polyphasic motor unit action potentials are intermixed with the larger ones, and rapid recruitment is seen in some areas. Clinical presentation generally provides compelling evidence to suggest a primary myopathy in this setting.

Spontaneous activity

Due to changes in acetylcholine receptors, the denervated muscle fibres become hyperexcitable and spontaneously discharge, seen on needle EMG as fibrillation potentials and positive sharp waves. **Fasciculation potentials** are also common, whereas **myokymia**, **neuromyotonia**, and other spontaneous activity are relatively unusual, but may give a clue to the underlying aetiology in certain circumstances.

Motor unit action potential morphology

In partial axonal lesions, unaffected motor axons sprout extra terminal nerve branches over a period of weeks and months. They supply nearby denervated muscle fibres, resulting in abnormally large motor units. On EMG this is reflected in long-duration motor unit action potentials which are high amplitude and polyphasic. Note that it is the surviving, comparatively healthy, motor units that are seen on EMG.

Recruitment and interference patterns

With gentle muscle contraction large motor units are recruited sooner than they would usually be, reflecting both the reduced number of motor units and their abnormally large size in a partially denervated muscle. Thus, rather than

Table 6.2 Neurogenic and myopathic EMG findings. Note that the table necessarily represents a generalization from which there are some exceptions

	Normal	Neurogenic	Myopathic
Spontaneous activity	None (except at end plate)	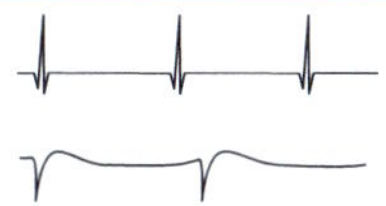 Fibrillation potentials and positive sharp waves if there is ongoing remodelling of motor units, plus fasciculations	Often none, but may have fibrillations and positive sharp waves
Motor unit action potential	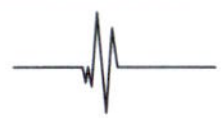	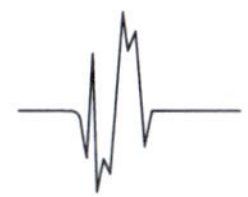	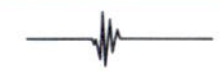
Duration	N	↑	↓
Amplitude	N	↑	↓
Phases	N	↑	↑
Recruitment	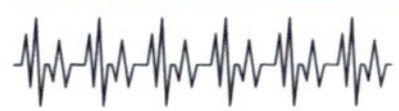 N (orderly recruitment of successively larger motor units)	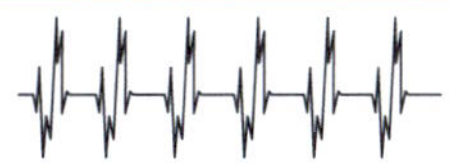 Reduced (few motor units activated, they fire at high rates in relative isolation)	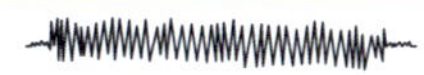 Rapid (many small motor units activated with weak contraction)
Interference pattern	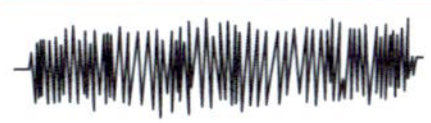 N, Full	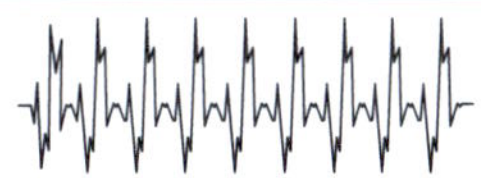 Reduced (discrete large potentials still seen and heard at maximal effort, and the muscle is weak)	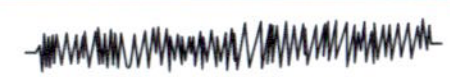 Full (but low amplitude, and with a weak contraction)

N, normal; ↓, decreased; ↑, increased.

the usual pattern of small motor units being recruited first, an abnormally broad polyphasic motor unit action potential fires during weak contraction. As the force of contraction is increased there are fewer motor units to recruit, thus the unit already recruited fires faster and faster but in relative isolation—reduced recruitment. The interference pattern with maximal contraction is correspondingly reduced.

Myopathic EMG

Spontaneous activity

It is not uncommon to see fibrillation potentials and positive sharp waves in a myopathic condition, especially if it is necrotizing. It is believed that damage to terminal axons or splitting of muscle fibres causes intramuscular denervation, and therefore hypersensitivity and spontaneous fibrillation potentials. The important point is that fibrillations and positive sharp waves do not necessarily imply primary nerve pathology. Myotonic discharges might be seen, and can give a clue to the underlying condition. Complex repetitive discharges are sometimes seen in chronic myopathies.

Motor unit action potential morphology

In myopathic conditions most motor units contain fewer muscle fibres than normal, and as a result the motor unit action potentials tend to be short duration, low amplitude, and polyphasic. However, some relatively long-duration, high-amplitude motor unit action potentials may be intermixed as a result of reinnervation following muscle fibre splitting or degeneration of intramuscular terminal motor axons. It takes at least several weeks for such motor unit remodelling. In this context, large motor unit action potentials do not imply an additional neuropathic process. Note also, that short-duration polyphasic motor unit potentials are not specific to myopathies, and can be seen with reinnervation after axonal pathology, discussed later in this section.

Recruitment and interference patterns

With weak contraction of the muscle more motor unit action potentials fire than normal since they are small and individually so weak. This early/rapid recruitment means it may be almost impossible to see individual motor unit action potentials on EMG. Despite a weak contraction the interference pattern is full, but it tends to be of low amplitude, reflecting the small motor units.

Conduction block

Peripheral nerve conduction block may occur in isolation, without axonal damage that would result in Wallerian degeneration. The motor axon retains normal contact with muscle fibres, so there is no EMG evidence of spontaneous activity, and the motor unit action potentials remain normal. With minimal contraction there are essentially normal units recruited (in some settings they may be rather bigger than expected depending on how many, and what types of nerve fibre have been blocked). As the subject tries to increase the force of contraction partial conduction block limits the number of motor units that can be recruited ('reduced recruitment'), so the muscle is weak. However, since central drive remains good the available units fire at very high rates but achieve only a reduced interference pattern (see Table 6.3).

Upper motor neuron lesion

With upper motor neuron lesions the ability to recruit and drive the intact lower motor neurons is impaired. On EMG there is characteristically no spontaneous activity, and motor unit action potentials have normal morphology. With weak activation there are a normal number of motor units recruited appropriately. However, despite maximal effort the muscle remains weak and

Table 6.3 EMG patterns with conduction block, central pathology, or abnormal neuromuscular transmission. Note that the table necessarily represents a generalization from which there are some exceptions

		Peripheral conduction block (partial)	**Central loss of drive (upper motor neuron lesion, pain, volitional)**	**Neuromuscular junction**
Spontaneous activity		None	None	None (unless severe, as in botulism)
Motor unit action potential	Duration	N	N	N (↓ if severe)
	Amplitude	N	N	N (↓ if severe)
	Phases	N	N	N (↑ if severe)
Recruitment		Reduced. High firing rate due to preserved central drive, but block prevents recruitment	Poor activation. Normal firing rates but failure to recruit more than a few units	N usually. If severe, looks like a myopathy, with rapid recruitment
Interference pattern		Reduced	Reduced	N usually

N, normal; ↓, decreased; ↑, increased.

the lack of central drive prevents units firing at high rates or the recruitment of further motor units. The recruitment pattern is described as 'poor activation' due to poor central drive, and the interference pattern is reduced. Although in conduction block the interference pattern is reduced, the EMG findings are different since in that situation there is normal central drive, so few units fire at high rates (recruitment patterns are reviewed in Chapter 5).

EMG does not distinguish a loss of central drive due to an upper motor neuron lesion compared to reduced effort in response to pain or lack of volition.

Neuromuscular junction failure

Many cases of myasthenia gravis are relatively mild, and routine EMG remains normal or near normal with standard visual inspection. However, with persistent block of neuromuscular junctions, as in botulism or severe myasthenia gravis, fibrillation potentials may be seen, and motor unit action potentials can appear polyphasic and of short duration due to the functional loss of muscle fibres—the EMG appearances resemble a myopathy. There is generally some instability of the motor unit action potential from one activation to the next, reflecting intermittent blocking of the neuromuscular junction to a proportion of the muscle fibres. This is discussed further in Chapter 9.

Reinnervation findings

Following severe axonal injury to a nerve there will be slow regrowth of axons from the stump provided the endoneurium remains intact, the time course of which is considered in Chapter 8. When a regenerating motor axon reaches its target a small number of muscle fibres are initially innervated, and the subsequent 'nascent' motor unit action potentials are polyphasic and low amplitude, often with late 'satellite components'. Superficially they bear some resemblance to small myopathic units, but of course they occur in a completely different clinical context, and with increased effort there is a failure to recruit more motor units, in stark contrast to a myopathic muscle. Once again the wider electrophysiological and clinical context makes the diagnosis clear.

Over time, the small polyphasic units tend to become larger with the innervation of more muscle fibres. Furthermore, the recruitment pattern improves as more axons regrow, and fibrillation potentials become less frequent as muscle fibres are either reinnervated or cease to be electrically active.

Overview: What is the Pathology?

The electrodiagnostic findings expected with disease at different sites along the neuromuscular axis are summarized in Fig. 6.1 and Table 6.4. These

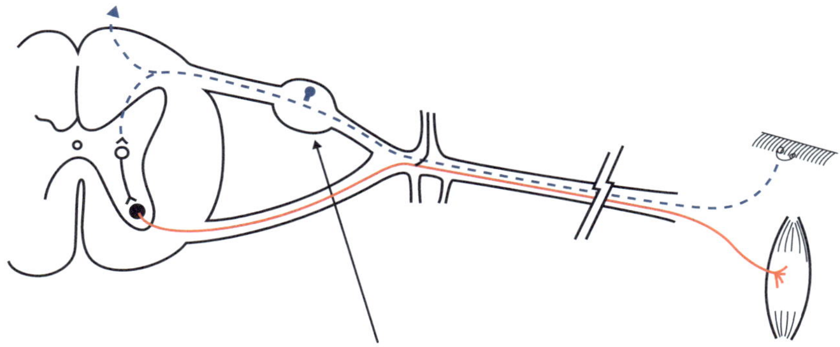

	Upper motor neuron	Anterior horn	Motor root	Dorsal root ganglion	Plexus	Nerve	Neuro-muscular junction	Muscle
SNAP	N 'preganglionic' ↔			Absent	↓ or absent ↔ If axon loss		N ↔	
CMAP	N	N or ↓ ↔ if very severe		N	↓ or absent ↔ (look at CV) (look for block)		N usually ↔ ↓ in LEMS	↓ if severe
EMG	N MUAPs ↓ central drive	Neurogenic ↔		N	Neurogenic if axon loss ↔		N usually	Myopathic

Figure 6.1 Pathology is determined by looking for patterns of nerve conduction and EMG findings. CMAP, compound muscle action potential; CV, conduction velocity; LEMS, Lambert–Eaton myasthenic syndrome; MUAP, motor unit action potential; N, normal; SNAP, sensory nerve action potential; UMN, upper motor neuron.

Table 6.4 Summary of neurogenic and myopathic EMG findings

	Neurogenic	Myopathic
Spontaneous activity	Fibrillations usually	Nil usually, sometimes fibrillations
MUAP morphology	Long duration High amplitude Polyphasic	Short duration Low amplitude Polyphasic
Recruitment	Reduced—few large units recruited	Rapid—early recruitment of many small units
Interference pattern	Reduced	Full (low amplitude)

changes reflect those expected at least several weeks after disease onset, and not necessarily those in the acute or very chronic setting. In trying to highlight the basic principles of how the neurophysiologist determines pathology it is inevitable that there are exceptions to some generalizations. Pathology, and therefore neurophysiological findings, evolve over time, and since this is critical to understand it is considered separately in Chapter 8.

It is worth highlighting the following general points since they help in understanding and interpreting neurophysiological studies:

- The amplitude of sensory responses is only reduced with pathology at or distal to the dorsal root ganglion ('**postganglionic**') resulting in axon loss. Thus sensory potentials would be expected to be normal in radiculopathies or motor neuron disease. Furthermore they would also remain normal with demyelinating lesions that lie proximal to both stimulation and recording sites.
- A marked reduction in motor response amplitude (CMAP) commonly reflects axonal pathology along the motor nerves—a neuropathy of some sort, either focal or generalized. Proximal pathology at the anterior horn cell and motor root has to be very severe at more than one root level before there is a severe reduction in the CMAP. Likewise, distal pathology at the neuromuscular junction or muscle is rarely sufficient to cause a severe reduction in CMAP amplitude (although the Lambert–Eaton myasthenic syndrome is an exception, considered further in Chapter 9).
- A neurogenic pattern of EMG findings is seen with pathology anywhere along the course of the motor neuron that results in **axonal degeneration**, whereas a myopathic pattern of EMG findings is specific to muscle. Remember that EMG can record a few large motor unit action potentials amongst the smaller myopathic ones in chronic myopathies. Also, following severe axonal injury new regenerating motor unit action potentials may be small and polyphasic. Thus the morphology of motor unit action potentials is not specific to a single pathology despite common descriptions of the units being 'myopathic-looking' or 'neurogenic-looking'. The key to correct diagnosis comes from the wider pattern of EMG findings and the clinical context.

Chapter 7

Axis 2: Localization

Key points

- The distribution, not just the type, of pathology requires special attention in the diagnosis of most conditions, for example, mononeuritis multiplex, motor neuron disease, and myopathies.
- Sometimes precise localization of pathology is impossible. This depends on the type and location of pathology, and the timing of the electrodiagnostic examination.
- Two factors determine disease severity: the degree to which a region is affected, and the extent of spread beyond that single region (localization).
- Focal axonal lesions are generally localized by EMG, not nerve conduction, but the ability to do so may be limited by the number of branches from the nerve, and whether pathology is fascicular.
- Conduction block may be localized by short-segment nerve conduction studies, sometimes called 'inching'.
- The amplitude and area of sensory or motor responses provide a reasonable estimate of the amount of axon loss, provided there is no demyelination causing either temporal dispersion or conduction block.
- The neurophysiological examination should be stopped once the referral question is answered or the patient is uncomfortable, or if further tests will add little further information.

From clinical and subsequent neurophysiological assessment of the type of pathology present (Chapter 6), the electromyographer goes a long way towards determining the location of that pathology along the longitudinal (brain to muscle) neuraxis. In other words, it usually rapidly becomes apparent that the disease process is **preganglionic**, or affects the left ulnar nerve, the neuromuscular junction, or the muscle itself.

This chapter considers situations in which special efforts are made to take localization a step further. This is conceptually slightly different to simply determining the type of pathology, and is important since it frequently dictates the extent and duration of the neurophysiological examination. The localization of pathology may be considered in two directions:

1. *Longitudinal localization*. Sometimes particular effort is made to locate the site of pathology along the nerve or at another location between brain and muscle. For example, accurate longitudinal localization can help determine the best treatment of focal compression neuropathies, or may help gauge severity of a length-dependent generalized polyneuropathy.
2. *Transverse localization*. The neurophysiologist carefully considers the spread, or distribution, of pathology within a region or to other regions of the body. For example, it is important to know whether EMG evidence of denervation is focal or widespread in order to diagnose motor neuron disease. It can also be very helpful to know the distribution of myopathic change, whether a neuropathy is focal or part of a mononeuritis multiplex, or whether a disease process has affected just one trunk or the whole of the brachial plexus.

Disease severity is considered together with localization since the severity of a pathological process depends not only on the degree to which a single area is affected, but also how widely distributed the process is. Severity of disease becomes apparent to the electrophysiologist whilst performing tests to localize pathology, but deserves special attention and comment since the severity of disease may play an important role in prognosis and management. Neurophysiological tests are relatively good at determining the extent or spread of disease, but quantification of severity in a single area can be difficult, and sometimes uses techniques beyond the scope of this text.

What You Need to Know Before You Localize

Interpretation of the neurophysiological examination requires a good deal of background knowledge, most of it clinical neurology. It is essential to understand how neurological disease presents and is likely to progress, for example, the distal rather than proximal weakness in certain myopathies, the expected findings in a mononeuritis multiplex compared to a length-dependent polyneuropathy, and so on. There are many excellent neurology texts the reader can refer to for this. In addition, reasonable knowledge of peripheral nerve anatomy and examination is essential, and the 'Anatomy Buster' section of this book should help with this (Chapter 13).

Armed with this background knowledge the referring clinician and examining neurophysiologist must be clear about the aim of the examination. For example, if the patient is known to have inclusion body myositis but the clinically important question is why they have new-onset left wrist drop, this must be clear from the request. The neurophysiologist must perform a clinical neurological examination tailored to the referral question, since this will influence which muscles and nerves are tested, and reduce the likelihood of misinterpretation of results. Finally, factors likely to limit the extent of the neurophysiological examination should be borne in mind, such as cooperation in very young or confused patients, or accessibility in patients with dressings on the intensive care unit.

Longitudinal Localization: Focal Neuropathies

It is common to use nerve conduction and EMG to localize and characterise focal neuropathies. The technique employed will depend on the type of pathology.

Focal demyelination

When demyelination causes conduction block, the approximate location of the lesion will be apparent on routine nerve conduction studies provided it lies between the stimulating and recording electrodes (Chapter 3). In some settings a more precise location can be identified by short-segment studies, sometimes known as '**inching**' (Fig. 7.1). With this technique the site of stimulation is gradually moved distally in measured 1–2cm increments from a starting point proximal to the region of block. Because of conduction block the distal CMAP will be small at the proximal starting point. Successive stimuli are delivered, and the site of block is identified just proximal to the stimulating cathode at the point at which the CMAP amplitude returns to normal, implying that at this point the cathode lies just beyond the region of block. A jump in latency is also generally apparent due to slowing of conduction through the region of block.

Inching is a moderately time-consuming technique, and to be accurate relies on the pathology being focal plus the nerve being relatively superficial, and its course well defined. If the nerve is deep and high-intensity stimulation is required, there is the likelihood of nerve excitation distant from the cathode, reducing the accuracy of the technique.

Focal axonal lesions

Routine nerve conduction studies cannot accurately localize an axonal lesion even if it is focal since the lesioned axons make no contribution to the CMAP

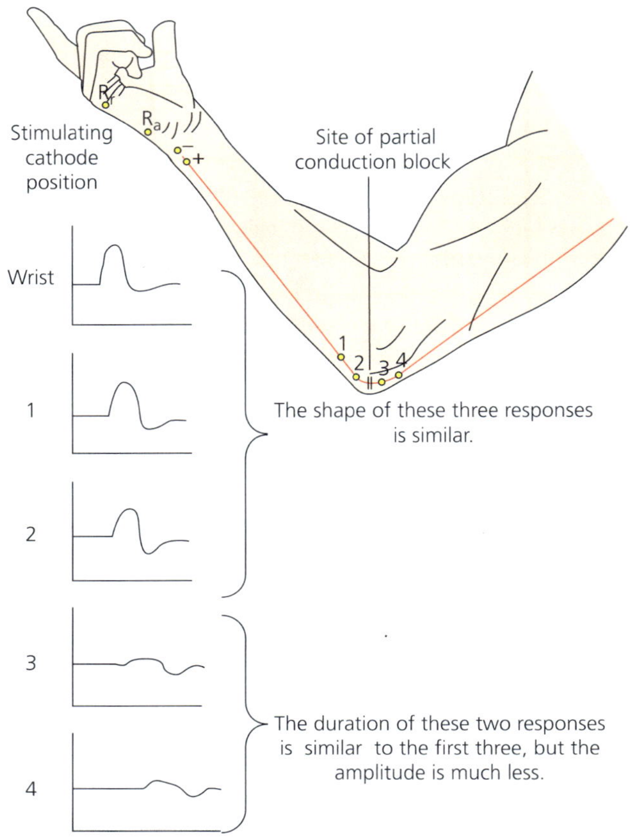

Figure 7.1 Focal neuropathies: localization of partial motor conduction block in the ulnar nerve by short-segment stimulation.

with stimulation either above or below the site of pathology. In axonal lesions the CMAP does not decrease with stimulation proximal to the lesion as it would in conduction block. The one exception is very acute lesions which are just a couple of days old in which an apparent conduction block pattern may be seen before Wallerian degeneration is complete (see Chapter 8).

In general, needle EMG can help localize focal axonal lesions according to the pattern of muscles denervated. However, accurate localization with this technique relies on the lesion occurring at a site where the nerve gives off many branches to muscles, both proximal and distal to the site of pathology. Unfortunately this is not always the case, and many nerves go a considerable distance without branch points, for example, the ulnar nerve proximal to the elbow. Furthermore, the accuracy of localization will be compromised when the lesion is patchy (fascicular) since some distal muscles may remain unaffected (see 'Type of nerve pathology' section)

Transverse Localization: When to Stop

In principle, localization is easy. The neurophysiologist aims to test above and below the lesion in order to determine its extent, and to test nerves and muscles which would help disprove important differential diagnoses. To strengthen conclusions some internal consistency of findings is desirable, for example, in a **radiculopathy** denervation is ideally detected in more than one muscle supplied by a particular nerve root.

But there is always another muscle or nerve that can be tested to determine spread, or transverse localization, of disease. In a quest to be thorough it is important to know when to stop. To some extent this is determined by the context in which the electromyographer works and whether the referring clinician sends only patients with clinically definite neuromuscular problems (for confirmation) or sends patients with more subtle or unexplained symptoms. It helps if the referring clinician is aware of factors that will limit the examination:

1. Examination is stopped once the referring clinician's specific question is answered unless there is a good reason to continue.
2. Particular attention is paid to patient discomfort. The most robust and discriminatory tests are performed first, particularly in paediatric practice.
3. It is sometimes impossible to be definite about localization, even if more and more tests are performed, since pathology can be patchy and there are slight variations in normal anatomy. Extensive testing of unlikely hypotheses will increase the incidence of false positives.

Consider two contrasting clinical examples:

- *Case 1.* A 62-year-old man was referred with suspected early amyotrophic lateral sclerosis, but the clinical diagnosis remained insecure, and there was prominent hand weakness raising the possibility of multifocal motor neuropathy with conduction block. Extensive nerve conduction studies were performed to look for evidence of conduction block, including proximal nerve root stimulation, followed by extensive EMG to look for evidence of widespread subclinical denervation. Such an extensive study, possibly with a follow-up study too, is justified in order to help try and make a definitive early diagnosis, thus determining prognosis and influencing treatment.

- *Case 2.* An adopted 8-year-old boy was referred because of a suspected genetic demyelinating neuropathy. In this context the single most useful neurophysiological test is likely to be motor conduction, therefore the first nerve the electrophysiologist tested was motor conduction in the median nerve in the forearm. This revealed severe slowing (19m/s), with relatively preserved amplitude and no significant dispersion or conduction block. The child became upset, and the clinical suspicion had been confirmed, therefore little was lost by avoiding further testing at this stage in favour of genetic tests.

Problems with localization

There are a number of settings in which the standard nerve conduction and EMG examination may fail to localize focal pathology. This may relate to the type of nerve pathology, its site, or the timing of neurophysiological examination in relation to injury. Some are considered in more detail in Chapter 10.

Type of nerve pathology

Consider first the effect of type of nerve damage with the example included earlier of an ulnar neuropathy at the elbow. Most have some demyelination, so may be localized because of conduction slowing or block. However, if there is purely axon loss the lesion cannot be localized by nerve conduction testing, and although EMG may help by finding denervation in muscles distal to the lesion, there are long sections of the ulnar nerve without branches to muscles in which precise EMG localization would not be possible. Furthermore, pathology may be patchy, and only involve certain fascicles of a nerve, sparing some muscles distal to the lesion which would therefore be 'false localizing' on EMG.

There are many examples in which axonal pathology is commonly patchy, including motor radiculopathies and stretch lesions of the sciatic nerve. The latter often preferentially involves peroneal fibres and the neurophysiological assessment may appear more like a common peroneal neuropathy at the fibular head (albeit without evidence of focal demyelination) unless there is also denervation of the short head of biceps femoris, which is innervated by a branch of the peroneal nerve proximal to the fibula head.

Site of pathology

The site of nerve pathology will of course affect how well it can be detected and localized since some regions of the peripheral nervous system are relatively inaccessible to testing. For example, the lower sacral nerves have neither sensory nor motor nerves that are readily accessible, and the S2–4 nerve roots provide little or no innervation to the limb muscles commonly assessed with EMG. This renders the routine neurophysiological examination insensitive to pathology in this region. Another example is proximal nerve root demyelination, which may pass undetected since there is no denervation on EMG without axonal loss.

Timing of the examination

In some settings the ability of the neurophysiological examination to localize pathology may be affected by its timing.

For example, the electrophysiological distinction between L5/S1 root and lumbosacral plexus pathology relies to a large extent on the loss of superficial peroneal and sural sensory responses in the latter (indicating postganglionic pathology) but not the former. However, lower limb sensory responses may be undetectable because of oedema, dressings, or other factors. In this setting the finding of paraspinal muscle fibrillation potentials is helpful and favours root pathology, but there may only be a relatively brief window of opportunity to detect them. Paraspinal fibrillations tend to appear early in motor radiculopathies since the muscle is so near to the site of nerve injury. They may be present within a week or two of injury, but tend to disappear first with reinnervation, again since they are so proximal. There may therefore only be a relatively short window in which their presence can help localize pathology.

Another example in which timing of the electrodiagnostic examination affects our ability to localize pathology is following an acute partial axonal lesion. In the first few days post-injury, before Wallerian degeneration, the nerve conduction results appear similar to those expected in focal conduction block due to myelin dysfunction. A normal distal CMAP would be recorded following stimulation distal to the lesion (the nerve has not degenerated yet), but a reduced CMAP is seen with proximal stimulation—a conduction block pattern. The lesion could be localized by 'inching' as described earlier. However, within a week or two Wallerian degeneration will be near complete, and the CMAP will be small with both proximal and distal stimulation, thus the opportunity for localization by nerve conduction is lost (see Chapter 8 for further details of the timing of neurophysiological examination).

Disease Severity

Axonal pathology

In clinical practice the most commonly used estimate of the severity of axonal pathology is the reduction in amplitude or area of the motor or sensory responses. One problem is the relatively wide range of normal amplitudes in the population, so when a patient is studied for the first time there is no way of telling what their premorbid amplitude was, and therefore no way of knowing by how much it may have decreased. Side-to-side differences help to some extent, for example, a sural amplitude of 14uV in a 20-year-old may be in the normal range, but it is not normal if the unaffected contralateral response is 49uV.

Of course, with follow-up studies there is the benefit of reference back to the previous study, in which case CMAP changes can help gauge the severity and track the evolution of axonal pathology within the limits of reproducibility of the test. Another limiting factor, however, is the pathology itself, since there is a tendency for surviving motor axons to reinnervate denervated muscle fibres, forming large motor units. This is of course desirable in order to maintain strength, but in chronic axonal neuropathies it means that the CMAP amplitude may be an overestimate of the number of surviving motor axons. There are more complex neurophysiological techniques designed to study the number and size of motor units, but these are beyond the scope of this text. It should be recalled that CMAP amplitude reflects not only the number of axons but also the synchronicity of their firing, thus it is not specific for axon loss—a reduction in amplitude may result from patchy demyelination causing temporal dispersion, or from a number of technical factors.

In general, routine qualitative needle EMG is very sensitive at detecting axonal pathology, but less good at quantifying it. The problem is in part due to the selective sampling of the muscle inherent in needle EMG, such that patchy pathology can be missed. It is also due to the fact that mild denervation can appear similar to moderate disease, and may be reported in a similar way, such that from one test to the next the two cannot be distinguished.

Qualitative EMG does, however, still have a role in gauging the severity of neuromuscular disease. For example, after severe axonal lesions it is easy to tell apart the muscle with no functioning motor units from that with a couple of active motor units, and that with many active units. Such coarse distinctions should be relatively robust between studies and examiners, and they are clinically useful, for example, helping to guide the decision of whether to operate following traumatic nerve injury at a time when the clinical assessment may be extremely difficult.

EMG of course has a role in the assessment of disease severity by looking for spread to different regions rather than purely quantifying disease at a single site. EMG is particularly suited to this role since it is sensitive at detecting mild neurogenic change that may not be evident clinically.

Demyelinating pathology

The severity of demyelinating pathology can be assessed, to some extent, by the magnitude of reduction in conduction velocity. To enable this assessment the limb must be warm, since conduction velocity falls with nerve temperature. Very severe slowing, for example, upper limb motor conduction around 20m/s, is recorded in the context of severe demyelination, often found in hereditary demyelinating neuropathies.

The interpretation of sensory and motor response amplitudes may be complex in the context of demyelinating pathology. The CMAP amplitude does not provide a good measure of the amount of axon loss, as it does with pure axonal pathology, since amplitude is also reduced with conduction block and temporal dispersion. It is certainly possible for patchy demyelination to result in temporal dispersion with little reduction in conduction velocity (see Fig. 7.2), the clue being that duration of the response is prolonged. But also consider, for illustration, an unusual example in which a motor nerve is affected by an inflammatory neuropathy causing severe but fairly homogeneous slowing that results in little loss of response amplitude or temporal dispersion (Fig. 7.2b). If treatment then results in a patchy improvement in conduction velocity in some axons more than others it is possible that this may result in a paradoxical reduction in CMAP amplitude, despite the improvement in pathology, because of increased temporal dispersion. This is not generally seen, but with a good understanding of neurophysiology it might be suspected—the clue to the improvement is the increase in conduction velocity, although this may be small, and the relative preservation of response area suggests that despite the loss of amplitude there is little if any axon loss.

EMG may help in this setting by determining whether axon loss is contributing to the reduction in CMAP amplitude. The presence of secondary axon loss is important as it causes weakness and disability, and has implications for prognosis and treatment. However, it is common to have at least mild secondary axon loss with severe chronic demyelinating pathology, so it may prove difficult or impossible to detect a significant change in denervation with qualitative EMG alone.

In some situations there is a role for repeated nerve conduction, and sometimes EMG, in demyelinating neuropathies. For example, the degree of conduction block or slowing may help provide objective evidence about response to treatment or confirmation of disease progression. Similarly, evidence about disease spread and involvement of previously unaffected nerves helps assess disease severity. This can be particularly useful when clinical examination is

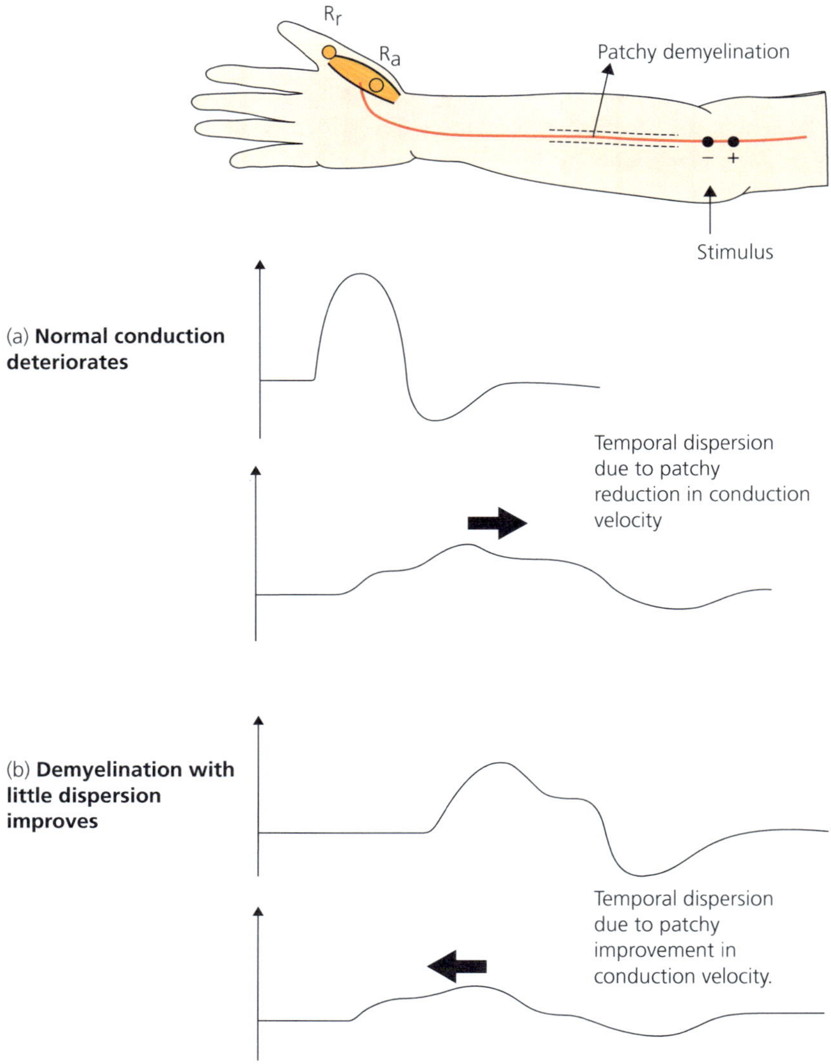

Figure 7.2 Assessment of the severity of demyelinating pathology: effects of temporal dispersion of responses.

difficult, or felt to be unreliable, and may help justify ongoing use of expensive therapy such as intravenous immunoglobulin.

Overview of basic aims of localization

An overview of basic neurophysiological findings which help localize pathology at different sites is provided in Table 7.1.

Table 7.1 Overview of neurophysiological localization of pathology, from brain to muscle. Look for internal consistency and test the longitudinal and transverse limits of the lesion

Site of pathology	Pattern of neurophysiological findings that help localization
Upper motor neuron	Sensory and motor conduction studies remain normal. EMG recruitment pattern may reflect poor activation but it is otherwise normal
Anterior horn cell	Neurophysiological findings are similar to motor radiculopathies (below) but in motor neuron disease the denervation is widespread. Extensive EMG sampling is required to look for evidence of denervation affecting different roots and nerves in the bulbar, cervical, thoracic, and lumbosacral regions. Proximal motor nerve stimulation may be needed to exclude motor conduction block, particularly with upper limb presentation
Motor nerve root	Normal sensory conduction confirms that pathology is likely to be preganglionic. Multiple muscles supplied by the same motor root show denervation despite the axons travelling via different peripheral nerves. Confirm whether there is denervation in muscles supplied by the nerve root above or below
Dorsal root ganglion	Commonly the pathology is widespread, resulting in reduction or absence of sensory responses that is not length dependent. Motor studies and EMG are normal
Plexus	Small sensory responses suggest there is postganglionic axon loss. However, abnormalities on nerve conduction studies and EMG do not follow the distribution of any single nerve or root. In the upper limb nerve conduction and EMG abnormalities can often localize the lesion provided the local anatomy is understood. Some plexus lesions can be patchy and hard to delineate, particularly in the lumbosacral region
Peripheral nerve	Pattern of nerve involvement is critical: is it one or many nerves that are affected, is it length dependent? Reduced distal sensory responses commonly suggest axon loss. With a weak, but not wasted, muscle proximal stimulation may identify focal motor conduction block. EMG shows denervation of muscles supplied by axons that traverse different motor roots but travel via the affected nerve

(Continued)

Table 7.1 (Continued)

Site of pathology	Pattern of neurophysiological findings that help localization
Neuromuscular junction	Myasthenia gravis may be focal, commonly ocular, or diffuse. Routine sensory and motor studies are normal, although motor amplitudes may be reduced in severe disease or with presynaptic pathology. Repetitive stimulation and EMG should be performed on a weak muscle. Routine EMG may be required to exclude denervation in a weak muscle with neuromuscular instability on single-fibre EMG. Usually rarer neuromuscular junction diseases have a distinct presentation
Muscle	Sensory and motor conduction is usually normal unless the myopathy is known to be associated with a neuropathy, or unless it is very severe when motor responses may be reduced. Test for characteristic patterns of muscle involvement: proximal, limb girdle, distal, facial weakness and so on. Type of spontaneous EMG activity may provide a clue to the diagnosis. Remember large 'neurogenic-looking' motor units may be seen in chronic myopathies

Chapter 8

Axis 3: Time Course

Key points

- Seddon's classification predicts prognosis and helps management of nerve injury. Axonotmesis refers to axonal discontinuity with the endoneurium intact—slow regrowth of axons is expected. With neurotmesis there is loss of continuity of axons and the endoneurium—no recovery is expected without surgical repair.
- Dividing an axon results in Wallerian degeneration of the distal axon, and an orderly sequence of neurophysiological findings. Early changes include loss of CMAP amplitude and appearance of fibrillation potentials on EMG.
- EMG performed even very early after nerve injury may help guide treatment—evidence of distal motor units under voluntary control proves the nerve is not completely sectioned, and may avoid early surgical intervention.
- In the first 2–3 weeks after nerve injury the neurophysiological examination does not accurately assess the severity, type or distribution of nerve damage. At this early stage partial axonal lesions may be difficult to tell apart from partial conduction block resulting from dysfunction of the myelin.
- Following axonal injury nerve regeneration starts with distal remodelling of surviving motor units (within weeks), and is followed by regrowth of axons from the site of injury (months usually). These changes are detected on needle EMG.
- In inflammatory myopathies disease activity can sometimes be estimated by EMG.

The timing of the neurophysiological examination in relation to nerve injury is critical since both nerve conduction and EMG findings change with the evolution of pathology. For the referring clinician this is important to understand since time from injury will affect interpretation, so the neurophysiological examination should be timed according to the clinical question to be answered. It is commonly believed that nerve conduction and EMG should only be performed late, at least a few weeks after nerve injury, but waiting is not always best, particularly when early surgery is considered, and some information may even be lost within a couple of weeks of injury.

Most important, and considered first here, is the sequence of nerve conduction and EMG changes that follow axonal injury and Wallerian degeneration of a nerve. Following this, it is also important to understand the expected neurophysiological findings as the nerve subsequently starts to regenerate, and to have some idea of the expected time course of change.

Evolution of pathology, and therefore neurophysiology, occurs not just in neuropathies, but in myopathic conditions too, so brief consideration is given to the evolution of EMG findings in inflammatory myopathies.

This chapter addresses temporal changes at a single site. Of course, the lateral spread of pathology over time to new nerves and muscles is important too, but is considered in Chapter 7 on the localization of pathology.

Acute Nerve Injury

Making sense of nerve conduction and EMG after acute peripheral nerve injury requires an understanding of how it is classified, in particular the work of Sir Herbert Seddon. By understanding the time course of Wallerian degeneration it becomes clear why some neurophysiological changes take several days to become apparent. It is important to appreciate that sensory and motor conduction studies will deteriorate at different rates, and that EMG fibrillation potentials may be absent for several days and will occur later in more distal muscles.

There are many pitfalls for the unwary: when examined within a week or so acute partial axonal lesions may be diagnosed as demyelinating because of apparent conduction block, or may be missed altogether. The key to avoiding such mistakes is to understand the expected sequence of neurophysiological findings in Wallerian degeneration, and to re-examine the patient.

Classification of peripheral nerve injury

In the 1940s, Seddon published a classification of peripheral nerve injury which matched nerve pathology to prognosis, thereby helping to manage patients, particularly those who might benefit from surgery (Table 8.1). Essentially, prognosis is good if conduction of action potentials is affected but axonal continuity is retained (**neurapraxia**). If the axon is disrupted but the endoneurium surrounding it is broadly intact (axonotmesis), recovery will

Table 8.1 Classification of nerve injury (after Seddon)

Pathology	Neurophysiology	Prognosis
Neurapraxia		
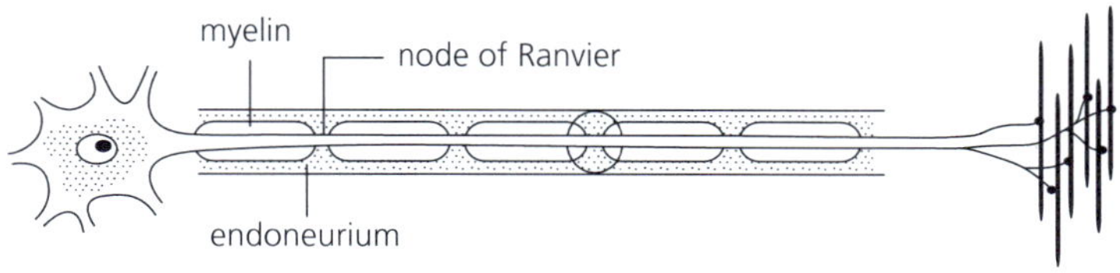		
Conduction block Dysfunction of the nodes of Ranvier causing failure of conduction. May be due to inflammation or compression. Structural nerve pathology not always evident	*NCS*: characteristically conduction block is seen. Also sometimes focal slowing and temporal dispersion. Normal responses with distal stimulation because there is no Wallerian degeneration. *EMG*: No spontaneous activity, normal motor unit action potentials but reduced recruitment and interference pattern	*Good, rapid recovery* In a normal subject a full recovery is usually made within about 2–3 months
Axonotmesis		
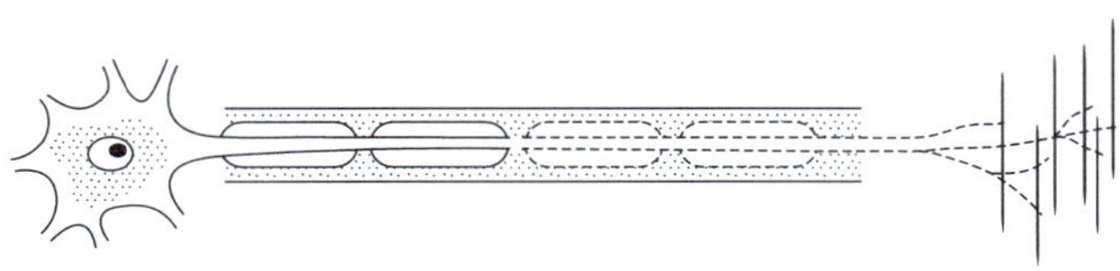		
Wallerian degeneration Axon continuity is lost, resulting in Wallerian degeneration distal to the lesion, with secondary myelin breakdown, shrinkage of the endoneurial tube and atrophy of denervated muscle fibres. Importantly the endoneurium remains mainly intact, so there is potential for axon regrowth, and therefore recovery	NB Findings depend on time after injury. After several weeks: *NCS*: the motor and sensory response amplitudes are small, but conduction velocity relatively preserved *EMG*: fibrillations, broad polyphasic motor unit action potentials but reduced recruitment and a reduced interference pattern	*Slow recovery* Recovery may only be partial, dependent on: (a) distal sprouting from any surviving motor axons, reinnervating muscle fibres (b) regrowth of severed axons provided the endoneurium is intact. Occurs at approximately 1mm/day.

(Continued)

Table 8.1 (Continued)

Pathology	Neurophysiology	Prognosis
Neurotmesis		
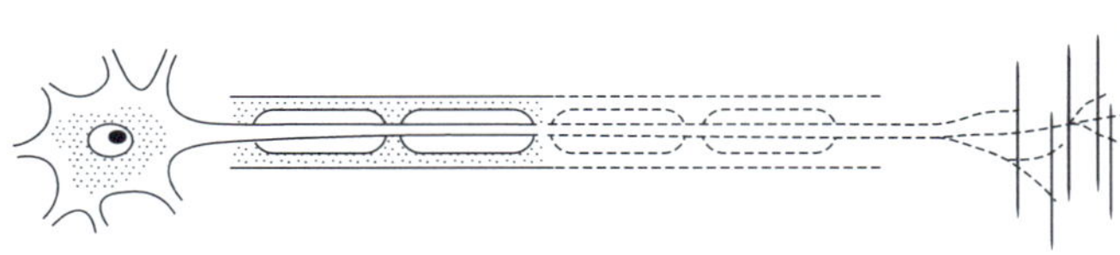		
Wallerian degeneration The axon and the endoneurium are completely severed. The discontinuity of the endoneurium means that axons fail to regrow as they have lost their usual guidance	Usually EMG and NCS indistinguishable from axonotmesis. (But the finding of even a single distal motor unit under voluntary control is important, implying there is not complete nerve transection)	*No recovery* Without surgical repair the complete loss of endoneurial integrity means regrowing axons lack direction and fail to contact the muscle. There is no significant regeneration

be prolonged because of the slow regrowth of axons at 1–2mm/day and distal remodelling of any surviving motor units. However, if both the axon and the surrounding connective tissue are severed (**neurotmesis**), there will be no significant regrowth of axons, and thus no recovery without surgical intervention.

It is common to experience mild nerve compression, with symptoms of heaviness, tingling, and sometimes numbness which resolve rapidly. This is probably caused by transient partial conduction block induced not by demyelination, but by ischaemia, with no structural change and therefore rapid resolution.

Pathological changes in Wallerian degeneration

When an axon is cut, the distal stump loses its connection to the cell body. As a result it gradually degenerates over a period of several days. The first change is failure of neuromuscular transmission, followed by breakdown of the axon. Schwann cells begin to catabolize the myelin and engulf axon fragments forming small ovoid compartments, termed myelin ovoids. Macrophages are recruited and contribute to the phagocytosis. The proximal nerve stump often shows degenerative changes generally affecting only the most distal two or three internodes before starting to regenerate. The cell body of the spinal motor neuron swells and production of proteins and RNA increases. Long after the disappearance of all neural constituents from the distal axon stump, a band of Schwann cells and collagen remains (band of von Büngner) which is the morphological substratum along which axons may regenerate.

The denervated muscle fibres downregulate their actin and myosin synthesis and decrease in size. There is resorption of myofibrils, but the cell remains viable, although not indefinitely. On pathological specimens these denervated muscle fibres have a small angulated cross section.

It is worth highlighting two points that have special relevance to the understanding of the associated neurophysiological changes:

- Synaptic transmission at the neuromuscular junction is lost relatively early, before degeneration of the distal axon.
- Neuromuscular transmission fails more rapidly if the axon is cut more distally. This may relate to the volume of the distal axon segment, and thus the supply of nutrients.

Neurophysiology and Wallerian degeneration

After transection the distal axon remains excitable for a few days before degenerating. It is convenient to divide the evolution of neurophysiological abnormalities into three phases following injury. It is worth stressing that the time course of neurophysiological changes depends on the length of the distal stump and diameter of the axon. With nerve lesions near to the target muscle the process will occur sooner than if the lesion is further away (Fig. 8.1).

Very early (approximately 0–3 days)

Initially both the motor and sensory response amplitudes will be normal, provided both stimulation and recording sites are distal to the lesion. There has been insufficient time for Wallerian degeneration. With stimulation proximal to the lesion, the amplitude recorded distally will be reduced in proportion to the degree of axon damage irrespective of the time from injury. In this situation the nerve conduction results will look the same as conduction block due to myelin dysfunction, with greater response amplitude following stimulation distal to the lesion compared to proximal. Of course if the lesion is very distal, near the recording electrode, the response amplitudes will be low at all stimulation sites since they are all proximal to the lesion, so the conduction block pattern is not seen.

EMG carried out within a couple of days of an acute axonal lesion will be too early to detect fibrillations. However, provided some axons in the nerve remain intact, EMG at this early stage will show normal motor unit action potentials firing at high rates, reflecting intact central drive, but reduced recruitment and interference pattern—in other words what appears to be a 'conduction block'

NCS	Approximate time, days	EMG
Normal sensory and motor conduction if both stimulation and recording is distal to the lesion. (stimulation proximal to the lesion will show 'conduction block' pattern acutely)	0–2	EMG appears as it would in conduction block: no spontaneous activity, normal motor unit action potentials firing at high rates but reduced recruitment and interference pattern
Decrease in CMAP amplitude starts about day 5, before a reduction in the sensory potentials	5	Fibrillations may appear as early as day 5–7 in muscles nearest the lesion
Sensory action potential amplitude begins to deteriorate about day 7. By about 10–14 days reduction of CMAP and sensory responses is complete	7–10 14	Fibrillation potentials in all denervated muscles, proximal and distal, by about 3 weeks
	21+	Surviving motor unit action potentials begin to become polyphasic at about 3–5 weeks, and eventually broaden as motor units remodel (months)

Figure 8.1 Neurophysiological changes with Wallerian degeneration. Note that the exact time course depends on the site of the lesion, with changes apparent earlier when the distance from the lesion to the muscle is short (CMAP, compound muscle action potential).

pattern (see 'Conduction block' section). If the lesion causes complete loss of axonal integrity the EMG will be silent, with no spontaneous or **voluntary activity**.

Intermediate (approximately 3–7 days)

After a few days there is progressive failure of the neuromuscular junction of transected motor axons. This precedes complete axon degeneration and results in reduction, or loss (depending on the degree of injury), of the CMAP a couple of days earlier than the sensory nerve action potential. In Wallerian degeneration the neuromuscular junction failure and axon loss precede demyelination, so conduction velocities remain relatively normal provided the CMAP or sensory action potential can be measured (Fig. 8.2). A small reduction in velocity may be seen when the responses are very small because of loss of the fastest conducting axons.

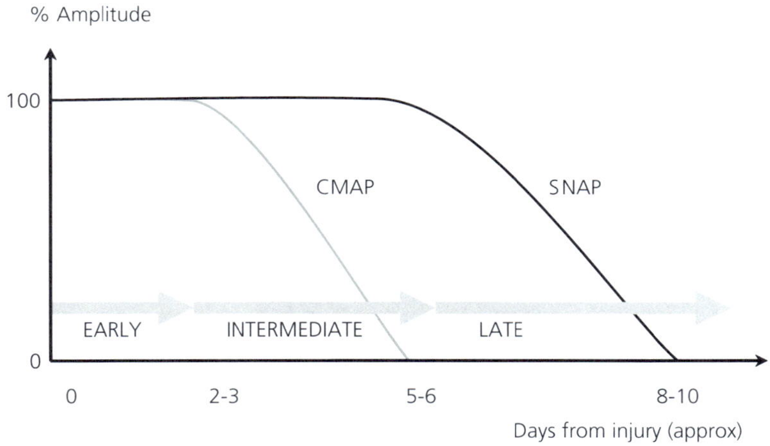

Figure 8.2 Motor responses are lost a few days before sensory responses in Wallerian degeneration. Time course depends on the length of the distal axon stump. CMAP, compound muscle action potential; SNAP, sensory nerve action potential.

In general there are no further EMG changes by this stage, it being too early to detect fibrillation potentials.

Later (beyond about 7 days)

By this stage the reduction in CMAP is generally complete, and if all axons were sectioned the CMAP will be absent, although the muscles innervated by the injured nerve will not yet be wasted. For a couple of days there may still be a small sensory response recordable, but following complete transection that soon will be lost too.

The EMG shows spontaneous fibrillation potentials, initially in muscles very near to the lesion at about 1–2 weeks post-injury, but in all muscles innervated by the injured nerve (even distal muscles) by about 3 weeks. At 3 weeks it is too soon for motor unit remodelling to be detected on EMG, so other than the appearance of fibrillation potentials and positive sharp waves the EMG remains similar to previously, with reduced recruitment of normal motor unit action potentials. The changes expected with subsequent motor unit remodelling and recovery are discussed in the section entitled 'Nerve regeneration after axonal injury'.

Conduction block: is pathology axonal or affecting myelin?

In the first few days after an acute axonal injury the nerve stump remains excitable, and a relatively normal response will be recorded distally provided stimulation is also distal to the lesion. With stimulation proximal to the lesion the response will be much smaller, and will resemble the neurophysiological findings in conduction block that is due to demyelination (sometimes termed 'dysmyelination' since very often the pathology causes dysfunction of the myelin rather than loss of myelin, thus explaining how recovery can be rapid) (Table 8.2).

Over time, the two pathologies, axonal versus dysmyelination, can easily be distinguished on neurophysiological grounds. Within 1–3 weeks following an axonal lesion, fibrillation potentials will be seen on EMG, initially in muscles close to the lesion site. None are seen in pure conduction block due to myelin dysfunction in the absence of axon loss. Also, by this stage any residual excitability of the distal separated axon stump will be lost, so the conduction block pattern of nerve conduction will no longer be present following axonal injury. The CMAP will be uniformly reduced, to a degree that reflects the severity of axonal damage.

Several weeks later, there will be EMG evidence of motor unit remodelling following a partial axonal lesion. The surviving motor units sprout new terminal axons to innervate neighbouring denervated muscle fibres, thus motor unit action potentials initially become polyphasic, and eventually become long duration and high amplitude. No such changes are seen if conduction block is secondary to myelin dysfunction. By 2–3 months it is common for dysmyelinating conduction block to have resolved. However, both nerve conduction and EMG abnormalities will remain following the axonal lesion, but by this stage they will be the expected findings of a chronic axonal lesion, with no evidence of conduction block.

When to request neurophysiology after acute nerve injury?

Early (0–2 weeks)

Neurophysiological examination within the first couple of days after traumatic nerve injury may help if there is a question of early surgical nerve repair. EMG can sometimes demonstrate motor units under voluntary control in a distal muscle which appears inactive clinically, implying that the nerve to that muscle cannot have been completely severed. With surviving motor axons across the lesion a non-surgical approach is often chosen, with the anticipation that regrowth of axons and remodelling of existing motor units will provide some recovery of function. Unfortunately the absence of voluntary EMG activity in weak muscles distal to the lesion is a less definitive finding. It does not prove that there has been complete transection of the nerve since there may be conduction block affecting some or all of the axons.

Table 8.2 Conduction block: focal dysmyelination or acute axonal pathology? Time refers to time elapsed following injury. Sensory nerve action potentials, SNAPs, are stimulated and recorded distal to the lesion

Time (approx. days)	Partial dysmyelinating conduction block		Partial axonal lesion	
	NCS (arrow indicates site of stimulation)	**EMG**	**NCS (arrow indicates site of stimulation)**	**EMG**
0–2	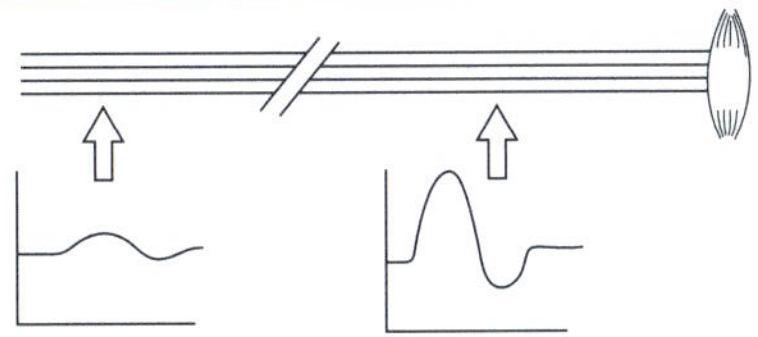 Proximal: ↓ CMAP Distal: full CMAP SNAP: normal	1. No spontaneous activity 2. Normal MUAPs 3. Reduced recruitment, high firing rate 4. ↓ interference pattern	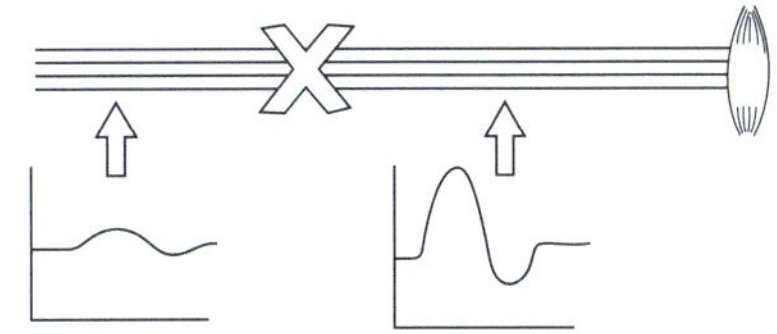 Proximal: ↓ CMAP Distal: full CMAP SNAP: normal	1. No spontaneous activity early 2. Normal MUAPs 3. Reduced recruitment, high firing rate 4. ↓ interference pattern
5–7	No change	No change	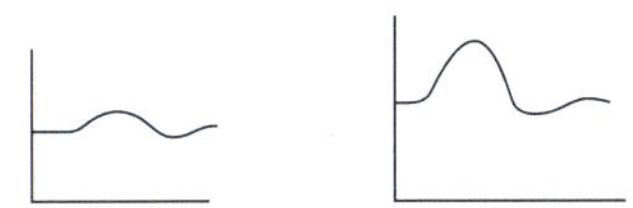 Proximal: ↓ CMAP Distal: slight ↓ CMAP SNAP: normal or minimally reduced	No change (too early for fibrillations in all but the most proximal muscles)

(Continued)

Table 8.2 (Continued)

Time (approx. days)	Partial dysmyelinating conduction block		Partial axonal lesion	
	NCS (arrow indicates site of stimulation)	EMG	NCS (arrow indicates site of stimulation)	EMG
>10	No change	No change	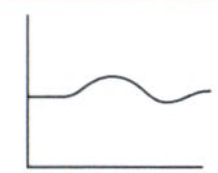 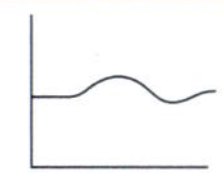 Prox: ↓ CMAP Distal: ↓ CMAP SNAP: small	Fibrillations by 3 weeks in all affected muscles Otherwise as above (too early for motor unit remodelling)
3 months later	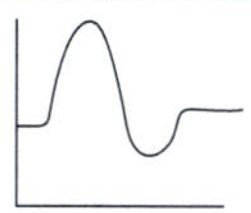 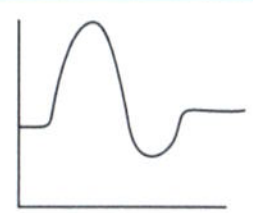 Proximal: full CMAP Distal: full CMAP SNAP: normal	Normal (recovery within 3 months usually)	No change (without significant axon regrowth/ remodelling)	1. May have fewer fibrillations 2. Some polyphasic, broad MUAPs and may be some nascent units in very proximal muscles 3. Reduced recruitment, high firing rate 4. ↓ interference pattern

CMAP, compound muscle action potential; MUAP, motor unit action potential.

Acute non-traumatic nerve injury is sometimes studied early in the disease course. For example, suspected Guillain–Barré syndrome is often confirmed by early neurophysiological examination even though findings at this stage can be subtle in comparison to disability (such as isolated loss of F-waves).

Some acute lesions, even pure axonal pathology, can be localized by the finding of apparent conduction block, which may be lost by about a week after injury if the pathology is axonal (see earlier and Table 8.2). However, it is relatively uncommon for this alone to justify an early neurophysiological assessment unless it will alter clinical management.

In the first week or two it is too early to reliably detect fibrillation potentials on EMG that might help localize or confirm axonal lesions, and too early to assess the severity of injury according to the loss of nerve conduction response amplitude, so consideration should be given to delaying or repeating the study a few weeks later.

Late (>3 weeks)

Waiting at least 3 weeks following injury will allow the site of the pathology to be localized according to the pattern of EMG denervation, and allow more reliable quantification of axon loss or other pathology since the CMAP and sensory action potential have stopped declining with Wallerian degeneration. Thus both severity and distribution of pathology are more reliably assessed late rather than early after nerve injury. Delaying neurophysiological examination of course makes sense if early assessment will not alter acute patient management. Furthermore it limits the need for repeated examination and use of emergency appointments, with obvious resource implications.

At times it is useful to perform repeat neurophysiological examination weeks or months after the initial injury. A common example is to see whether there are EMG signs of significant axon regeneration following severe nerve injury since this can guide the decision to perform further nerve or reconstructive surgery. In Guillain–Barré syndrome a repeat study may be required to confirm demyelination if a very early study was normal. Furthermore, it is sometimes helpful to determine whether there is substantial axon loss by the finding of spontaneous fibrillation potentials on EMG.

Nerve Regeneration after Axonal Injury

Provided the endoneurium remains intact to some extent, in other words injury has caused axonotmesis not neurotmesis, axons will start to regrow to reinnervated target muscles. This is a slow process and is generally preceded by distal remodelling and sprouting of any surviving motor axons to reinnervate nearby muscle fibres that have lost their nerve supply.

Weeks: distal motor unit remodelling

The remodelling of surviving motor units (if there are any) starts with sprouting of new terminal branches of motor axons to contact nearby denervated muscle fibres, thus increasing the size of surviving motor units. This distal reorganization occurs much earlier than any reinnervation resulting from regrowth of axons from the proximal stump at the site of the lesion. Since muscle fibre type is determined by the innervating neuron, the newly reinnervated muscle fibres assume the histochemical type of their neighbours. In this way the usual checkerboard pattern of fibre types seen at muscle biopsy is lost, and groups of contiguous myocytes are noted with the same histochemical type, termed 'fibre type grouping'.

With needle EMG these anatomical changes result in some motor unit action potentials becoming polyphasic, and unstable; that is, their morphology changes slightly each time they fire because of instability of neuromuscular transmission along the newly formed nerve sprouts. There is an abnormally high density of muscle fibres firing synchronously because of their common innervation (fibre type grouping), resulting in high-amplitude motor unit action potentials. As the process of axon sprouting and motor unit enlargement continues, the motor unit action potentials eventually become broader and high amplitude (Fig. 8.3).

Months: regrowth of motor axons

Provided the nerve injury did not completely section the endoneurium, regrowth of axons from the proximal nerve stump begins soon after injury and proceeds at about 1–2mm/day. The slowly advancing growth cone can be tracked clinically by tapping along the course of the nerve to elicit Tinel's sign. The first regenerating axons initially reinnervate just one or two muscle fibres in those muscles closest to the site of injury, but over time the size of the new motor units increases as more and more muscle fibres are contacted.

Needle EMG shows potentials sometimes termed 'nascent units'. These are new motor unit action potentials, which initially are very low amplitude and appear rather like a couple of time-locked fibrillation potentials, albeit under voluntary control, reflecting the initial innervation of just a couple of muscle fibres. With time, as more muscle fibres are innervated, the motor unit action potentials become increasingly polyphasic, but still often have 'satellite potentials'. These are small potentials which are time locked to, but distinct from, the main potential, reflecting the prolonged neuromuscular conduction time associated with new nerve sprouts. Over time, the number of fibrillation potentials decreases, in part because of reinnervation, but also because of a decline in activity of the muscle fibres that remain denervated. With chronic

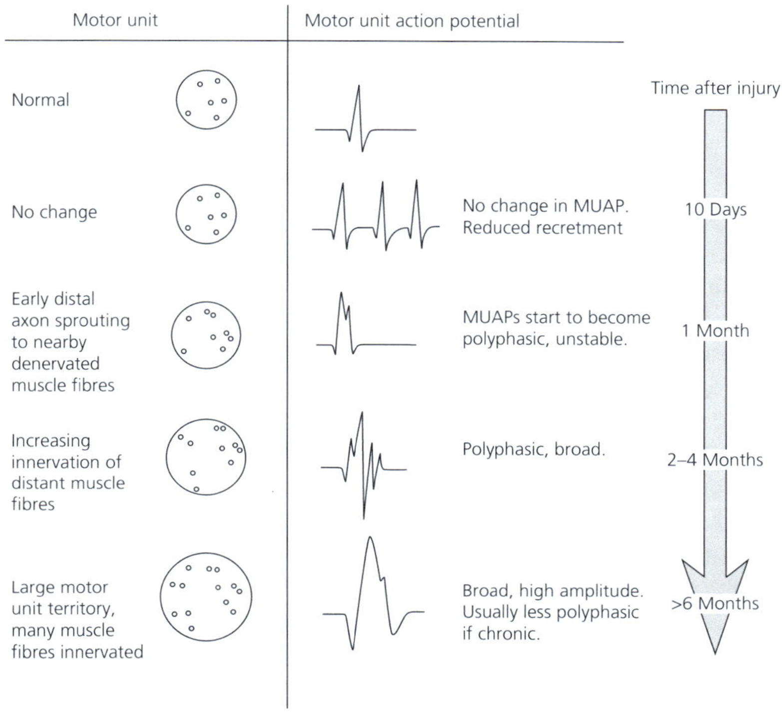

Figure 8.3 Motor unit action potential (MUAP) remodelling after partial axonal injury.

pathology the motor unit action potentials tend to become less polyphasic, but increasingly high amplitude and broad, reflecting the large size of surviving motor units.

The CMAP is slow to recover after a complete axonal injury, lagging well behind EMG changes since a reliable surface response generally requires several motor units to be functioning. Following such an injury a small CMAP may eventually become recordable, but sensory responses often remain undetectable. Note that with slowly progressive axonal pathology, such as might occur in motor neuron disease, the distal remodelling of motor units tends to preserve the CMAP amplitude, making it a less good marker of severity of axon loss. Specialized neurophysiological techniques which estimate the number and size of motor units can be used, but are beyond the scope of this book.

EMG and Inflammatory Myopathy

Over time, some myopathies undergo cycles of inflammation and disease activity followed by relative quiescence. The sequence of changes is less stereotyped

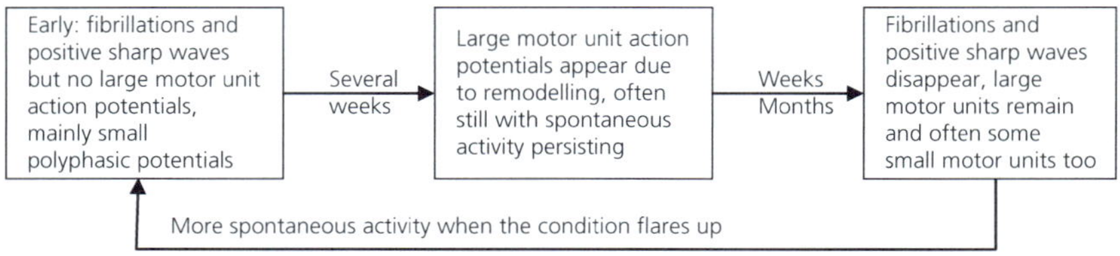

Figure 8.4 Evolution of EMG findings in inflammatory myopathies.

or predictable than those described after axonal nerve injury, but merits brief consideration since EMG may be of some help in determining the activity of inflammatory myopathies.

During their active phase, inflammatory myopathies tend to result in a reduced number of muscle fibres per motor unit, with some evidence of denervation of individual muscle fibres. This denervation is believed to result from intramuscular damage to small distal motor axons and muscle fibre splitting. On EMG the result is spontaneous fibrillation potentials and a myopathic EMG pattern where small polyphasic motor unit action potentials recruit rapidly with weak contraction to a full but low-amplitude interference pattern.

Once this active phase has passed there is a tendency for denervated muscle fibres to be reinnervated by sprouting of nearby motor axons. The result is that the EMG shows more longer-duration, higher-amplitude motor unit action potentials and fewer fibrillation potentials (Fig. 8.4). With a subsequent flare-up of disease the original EMG findings, particularly the fibrillation potentials, can recur.

In a patient with characteristic weakness, the EMG may of course play a role in diagnosing a myopathic process (reviewed in Chapter 6). However, in patients known to have an inflammatory myopathy such as polymyositis, treated with steroids, the EMG may give a clue to the likely aetiology of a deterioration whilst on treatment. In this setting the finding of profuse fibrillations and small polyphasic motor unit action potentials is suggestive of a flare-up of the underlying inflammatory myopathy, whereas an EMG without any spontaneous activity could be seen if the deterioration reflected a steroid-induced myopathy. Of course, this distinction cannot be made with absolute confidence from EMG alone, and there are other causes and investigations to consider.

Chapter 9

Special Studies of the Neuromuscular Junction

Key points

- To maximize the sensitivity of neurophysiological studies of neuromuscular transmission, a weak muscle should be tested in a warm environment.
- In health, the muscle end-plate potential generated following a nerve action potential is much greater than the threshold required to trigger a muscle action potential.
- Neither a decremental response to repetitive nerve stimulation, nor abnormally increased jitter on single-fibre EMG, is specific to myasthenia.
- Slow frequency (2–3Hz) repetitive nerve stimulation causes depletion of short-term acetylcholine stores, such that in myasthenics the minimum CMAP commonly occurs at stimulus four in a train: greater than 10% amplitude decrement is abnormal.
- The profile of the train of CMAPs elicited by repetitive stimulation, and their response to brief muscle contraction, helps confirm the diagnosis of myasthenia.
- Strong muscle contraction, or high-frequency nerve stimulation (painful), results in presynaptic accumulation of Ca^{2+}, thus increased acetylcholine release. In Lambert–Eaton myasthenic syndrome, this results in a large increase in CMAP amplitude.
- Single-fibre EMG (sfEMG) is very sensitive at detecting abnormalities of neuromuscular transmission. Stimulated sfEMG is useful in patients less able to cooperate.

The normal function of the neuromuscular junction is reviewed briefly in Chapter 1, and readers unfamiliar with the process should read this before continuing. This chapter considers how neuromuscular transmission can be

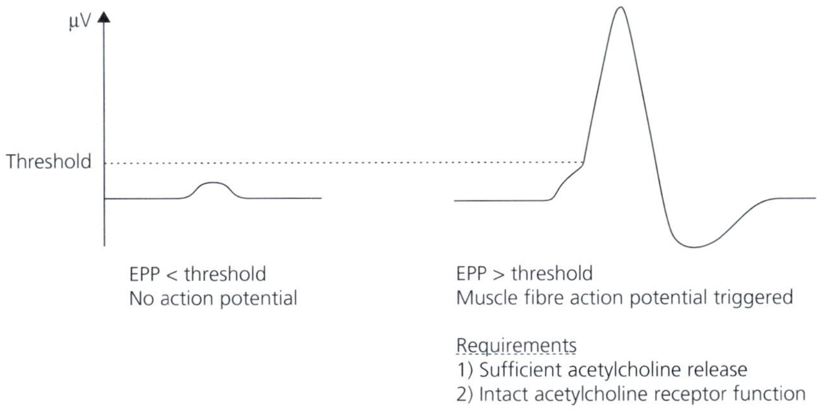

Figure 9.1 A muscle fibre action potential is generated provided end-plate potential exceeds threshold.
EPP, end-plate potential

tested by **repetitive nerve stimulation** and **single-fibre EMG** (sfEMG), and the results that might be expected with pre- and postsynaptic pathology.

Remember that the amount of acetylcholine released into the synaptic cleft will determine the end-plate potential, and this only results in a muscle fibre action potential if it reaches a certain threshold level of depolarization (see Fig. 9.1). The strength of muscle contraction and the amplitude of the CMAP are determined by the sum of many such muscle fibre action potentials.

In healthy muscle, the end-plate potential generated following neuromuscular transmission of an axonal action potential is much greater than the threshold required to trigger a muscle action potential—called the 'safety factor'. This is reduced in neuromuscular disease, resulting in failure of neuromuscular transmission at a proportion of junctions, and therefore weakness and potentially also a low-amplitude CMAP if disease is severe.

Repetitive Stimulation

Calcium and high-frequency stimulation (>10Hz)

A presynaptic influx of Ca^{2+} is required to package vesicles into the active zones and to release acetylcholine into the synaptic cleft. The influx of Ca^{2+} is rapid, via voltage-gated calcium channels, but it is pumped out over 100–200ms. Because of this relatively slow decrease in concentration, rapid electrical nerve stimulation (>10Hz) results in accumulation of Ca^{2+} in the presynaptic terminus. The slowly increasing presynaptic concentration of Ca^{2+} becomes the dominant factor affecting release of acetylcholine, and thus end-plate potential. Of course, in normal muscle this has little effect since all muscle fibres are activated anyway, so there is no increase possible, subtle changes relating to synchrony of firing of individual muscle fibres. However, when there is presynaptic neuromuscular junction failure, such as occurs in Lambert–Eaton myasthenic syndrome, high-frequency nerve stimulation progressively corrects the inadequate presynaptic concentration of Ca^{2+}, resulting in a dramatic increment in CMAP. This also explains the clinical finding of improved strength after forceful contraction.

Acetylcholine and low-frequency stimulation (2–3Hz)

With a rate of stimulation below about 5Hz there will be no progressive accumulation of Ca^{2+} in the presynaptic nerve terminus because of the rate at which it is removed. Thus at these frequencies there is no calcium-driven progressive potentiation of acetylcholine release. Acetylcholine is usually held in small amounts in active zone stores near the end plate. These are easily depleted, such that even at low rates of stimulation in normal muscle, the amount of acetylcholine released with each successive stimulus decreases for the first few shocks until active zone stores are replenished with secondary stores. In the normal situation, although this results in a slight dip in the end-plate potential generated, it still comfortably exceeds the threshold for muscle fibre activation due to the safety factor, and thus supramaximal nerve stimulation still results in a maximal CMAP after every stimulus (see Fig. 9.2). In diseases of the neuromuscular junction this dip in acetylcholine release is enough to result in failure of a proportion of the end-plate potentials to reach threshold, and thus failure of activation of some muscle fibres. The result is a decrementing CMAP with slow repetitive stimulation, especially on about the fourth stimulus, and a weak muscle.

The effect of muscle contraction on neuromuscular transmission

CMAP increment after brief contraction

Brief (10s) forceful muscle contraction is associated with high firing rates of motor units, up to 40–50Hz, resulting in the accumulation of presynaptic Ca^{2+} (see 'Calcium and high-frequency stimulation (>10Hz)' section), and therefore increased acetylcholine release. Thus, immediately after forceful brief contraction there is post-tetanic potentiation, with increased acetylcholine release and an increased end-plate potential. In myasthenia gravis this results in temporary repair of the decrement in CMAP seen with repetitive stimulation (see Fig. 9.3), and in Lambert–Eaton myasthenic syndrome this causes a dramatic increase in CMAP amplitude.

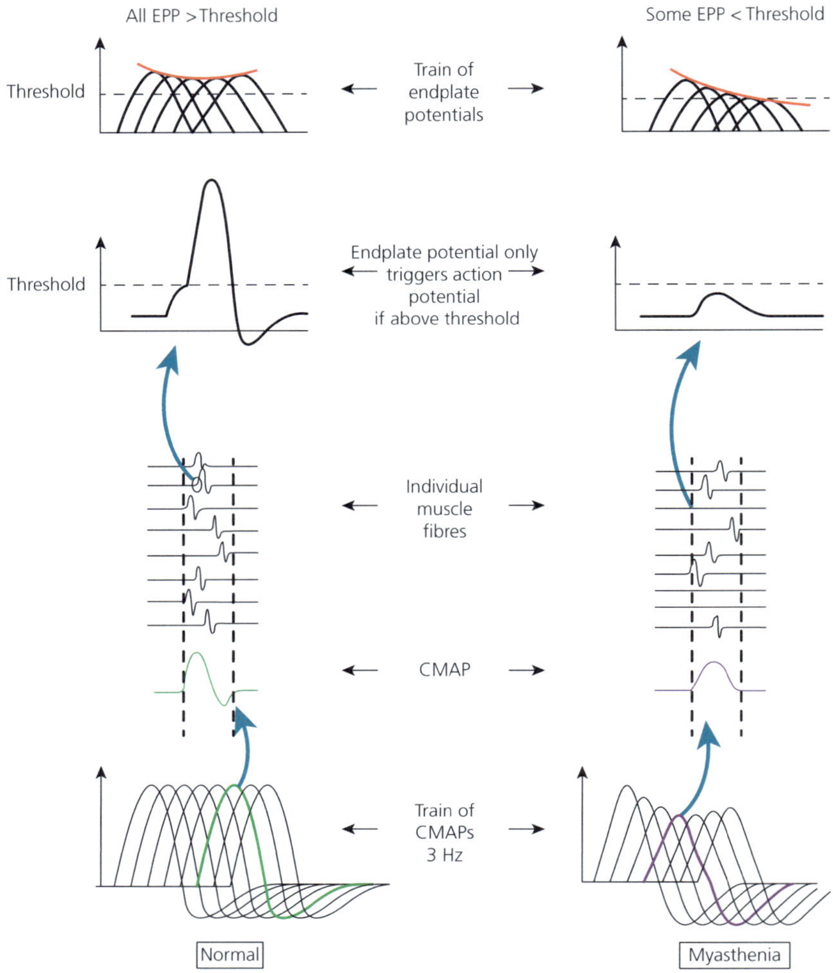

Figure 9.2 Low-frequency repetitive nerve stimulation. A slight dip in muscle end-plate potential results from depletion of active zone stores of acetylcholine during 3Hz repetitive stimulation, maximal at about the fourth stimulus. In normal muscle this does not result in failure to generate muscle fibre action potentials. In myasthenia the reduced safety factor means a proportion of muscle fibres may fail to be excited because the reduced endplate potential falls below threshold for triggering a muscle action potential. The result is a decremental CMAP response, usually with minimum amplitude by the fourth stimulus.

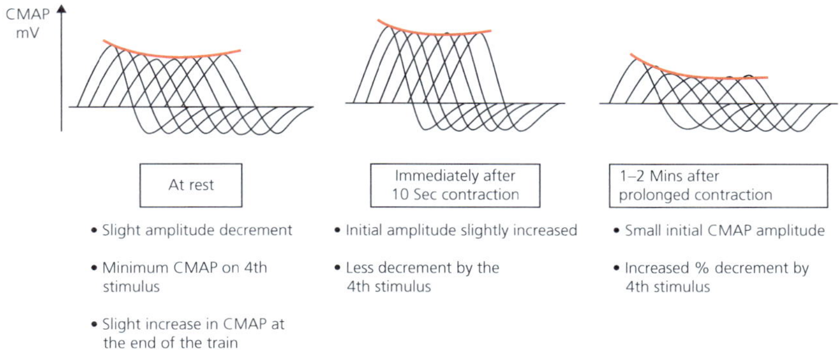

Figure 9.3 Effect of muscle contraction on repetitive stimulation in myasthenia: 1. Typical myasthenic CMAP decrement then mild late increment. 2. Improved immediately after brief contraction: both CMAP amplitude and percentage decrement. 3. Worsens with rest after prolonged contraction.

CMAP decrement following prolonged contraction

A minute or two after sustained forceful muscle contraction (for around 60s) there is no longer a high presynaptic Ca^{2+} concentration since there has been time for the concentration to drop. Furthermore, metabolic exhaustion probably plays a part in the reduction of acetylcholine released in response to a nerve action potential. In normal muscle the reduced end-plate potential still exceeds threshold due to the safety margin. However, in myasthenia the first CMAP of the train tends to be smaller than the original pre-exercise value, and the percentage decrement with repetitive stimulation is increased (see Fig. 9.3).

Repetitive stimulation in disease

Myasthenia gravis

The resting CMAP is usually nearly normal amplitude despite acetylcholine receptor blockade because of the safety factor, meaning that the end-plate potential still just exceeds threshold in almost all muscle fibres (except in very severe presentations). Slow repetitive stimulation at 2–3Hz causes a temporary dip in the amount of acetylcholine released from active zone stores as they become depleted prior to mobilization of larger stores. This, in combination with the receptor defect in myasthenia, causes the end-plate potential to drop below threshold for many muscle fibres, decreasing the CMAP: a decremental response to repetitive stimulation. This decremental response has a characteristic profile that is important to recognize. Most of the decrement occurs between the first and second stimuli, then the second and third and so on until the fourth or fifth response, after which there is a tendency for CMAP amplitude to increase slightly again (see Fig. 9.3 and Table 9.1).

If a similar train of ten stimuli at 2–3Hz is repeated immediately after 10s of forceful voluntary contraction the accumulation of presynaptic Ca^{2+} and subsequent increase in acetylcholine release tends to overcome the usual decremental response to stimulation: post-tetanic potentiation. This effect may be subtle and wears off quickly.

Table 9.1 Repetitive stimulation in diseases of the neuromuscular junction. Boxes indicate the key diagnostic tests

	Normal	**Postsynaptic (myasthenia gravis)**	**Presynaptic (LEMS)**
Single shock	1. 60–100 vesicles of ACh released per AP at one synapse 2. EPP >threshold 3. All muscle fibres activated 4. Full CMAP	1. Normal ACh release 2. EPP just >threshold in most or all fibres despite ACh receptor blockade 3. All, or most, muscle fibres activated 4. Full CMAP usually	1. ↓↓ ACh release due to lack of Ca^{2+} influx 2. EPP <threshold for most fibres 3. Few muscle fibres activated 4. Small CMAP
3Hz stimulation	1. ↓ in ACh release over first few shocks due to depletion of active zone store 2. EPP >threshold throughout, due to safety factor 3. All muscle fibres activated 4. Full constant CMAP	1. ↓ in ACh release over first few shocks 2. EPP <threshold in many fibres due to depleted and blocked ACh receptors 3. ↓ing number of muscle fibres activated over first few shocks 4. Dip in CMAP, minimum at 4/5th shocks (>10%)	1. ↓ in ACh release over first few shocks 2. EPP falls <threshold in even more fibres 3. Even fewer muscle fibres activated 4. CMAP shows decremental response, but difficult to detect from small start CMAP
Single shock immediately after 10–15s strong contraction (or tetanic stimulation—painful)	1. ↑ ACh release due to ↑ presynaptic Ca^{2+} and mobilization of long-term stores 2. ↑EPP 3. All fibres still activated 4 CMAP remains maximal	Similar to normal (left) in mild disease. Fast repetitive stimulation: the dip in CMAP characteristic with 2–3Hz stimulation does not occur because the ↑ Ca^{2+} causes ↑ ACh release (this is a short-lived effect)	1. ↑↑ ACh release due to ↑↑ presynaptic Ca^{2+} 2. ↑EPP 3. Many more fibres now activated 4. CMAP much bigger than the small pre-exercise value (>>50% usually, but the effect is short lived)

ACh, acetylcholine; AP, action potential; CMAP, compound muscle action potential, EPP, end-plate potential; LEMS, Lambert–Eaton myasthenic syndrome.

Criterion

During slow repetitive stimulation (2–3 Hz), greater than 10% decrement in CMAP amplitude from first to fourth response is abnormal.

Lambert–Eaton myasthenic syndrome

In Lambert–Eaton myasthenic syndrome the standard CMAP recorded after single-pulse stimulation is usually small because the arrival of a presynaptic action potential fails to trigger the usual degree of influx of calcium, thus less acetylcholine is released and the end-plate potential fails to exceed threshold in the majority of muscle fibres. Slow repetitive stimulation may elicit a dip in CMAP amplitude, but this may well be missed since the starting CMAP is so small. The most important electrophysiological test is post-tetanic potentiation. The increase in presynaptic Ca^{2+} immediately after a 10s forceful contraction causes a huge increase in acetylcholine release when a test shock is administered. The result is end-plate potential is increased, most muscle fibres are activated, and the CMAP increases—in Lambert–Eaton myasthenic syndrome the CMAP increase is commonly greater than 200%.

Criterion

After a 10s muscle contraction an increase in CMAP amplitude greater than 50% indicates significant post-tetanic potentiation.

Other disorders can affect neuromuscular transmission, with a resulting incremental response resembling that seen in Lambert–Eaton myasthenic syndrome. Examples include botulism, hypocalcaemia, hypomagnesaemia, and the toxic effect of some antibiotics and snake venom. In these cases the magnitude of the incremental response is usually less than that in Lambert–Eaton myasthenic syndrome. Electrophysiologists must watch out for 'pseudofacilitation' too, where a small increase in CMAP amplitude results from synchronization of muscle fibre firing in repetitive stimulation, but there is no increase in CMAP area.

Single-Fibre EMG

Using a standard, narrow-gauge, concentric EMG needle with appropriate filters, it is possible to compare the timing of activation of one muscle fibre to another from the same motor unit during gentle voluntary muscle contraction. The time difference between the activation of the two fibres is measured as the interpotential interval. Over a series of nerve action potentials the variation in this time interval between the two muscle fibres can be assessed, and is referred to as the 'jitter' (see Fig. 9.4). This variability is largely determined by variation in the time taken for neuromuscular transmission. This technique

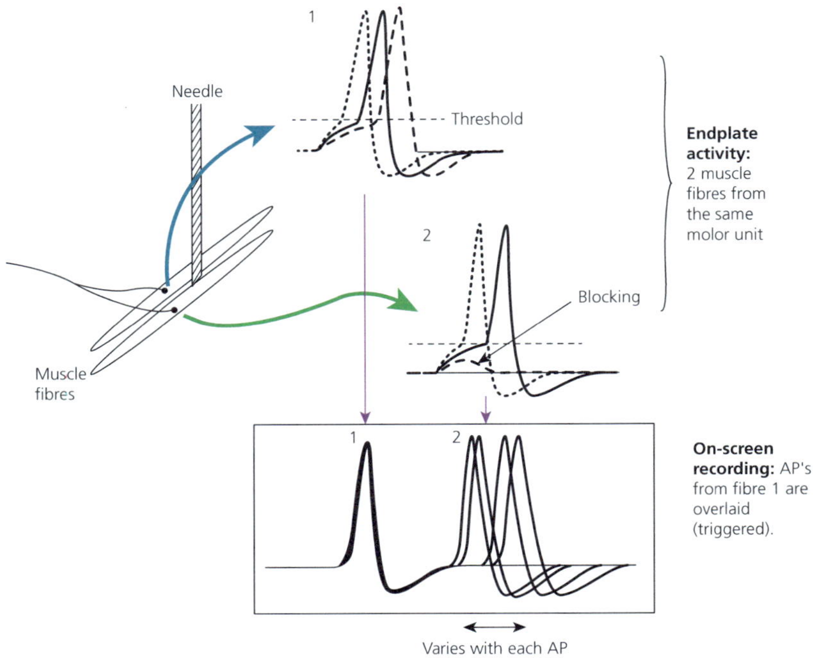

Figure 9.4 Single-fibre EMG. The needle records action potentials from two nearby muscle fibres in the same motor unit. The timing of activation of one relative to the other should be relatively stable—low jitter in normal muscle. In myasthenia there is increased variability, or jitter, and sometimes end-plate potential does not reach threshold, resulting in failure to trigger an action potential, termed blocking. The top two traces show end-plate depolarization in order to show blocking. The bottom trace shows what the electrophysiologist records, where action potentials from fibre one are displayed overlaid to emphasize the variability in interpotential interval, or jitter.
AP, action potential.

is called single-fibre EMG (sfEMG) since single muscle fibre action potentials are studied rather than the composite motor unit action potentials recorded in routine needle EMG.

Diseases of the neuromuscular junction, including myasthenia gravis, Lambert–Eaton myasthenic syndrome, and others, are characterized by increased variability in the time taken for neuromuscular transmission (resulting in increased 'jitter'), as well as occasional failure of transmission ('**blocking**'). When there is blocking, a proportion of the nerve action potentials only activate one rather than two muscle fibres—it is this, rather than increased jitter, that causes weakness.

Usually 100 sequential recordings are made of a particular pair of muscle fibres (takes only 20s if the nerve is firing at 5Hz), and 20 such pairs are recorded per muscle unless there is a definite abnormality detectable earlier. Jitter is usually expressed as the **mean consecutive difference** (MCD), a measure of the variability of the interpotential interval between the two muscle fibres, and is compared to muscle- and age-specific reference values. The mean of the MCDs from the 20 pairs is usually reported as well as the number of pairs with blocking or abnormally increased jitter.

Criterion

Abnormality is generally defined as either an increased overall mean MCD relative to controls, or two or more pairs with increased jitter or blocking even if the mean of 20 pairs lies within normal limits.

Stimulated single-fibre EMG

During voluntary sfEMG the patient is asked to maintain gentle contraction whilst the muscle is studied. This may be impossible in the intensive care unit or in young children since there is little patient cooperation. In this setting it is sometimes useful to test neuromuscular transmission by stimulating the nerve innervating the muscle directly, although it is still necessary for the patient to remain relatively still. It also allows for a change in the rate of stimulation, for example, in the Lambert–Eaton myasthenic syndrome a high rate of stimulation may result in reduced jitter due to accumulation of presynaptic Ca^{2+} enhancing acetylcholine release.

If stimulated sfEMG is performed, jitter represents the variability between stimulus onset (fixed) and time of activation of a single muscle fibre—only one neuromuscular junction is tested rather two in voluntary sfEMG. As a result normal stimulated sfEMG jitter values are lower than voluntary sfEMG, and a greater number of recordings must be made to be confident of detecting mild disease.

Maximizing the Sensitivity and Specificity of Tests of Neuromuscular Transmission

- Test the weakest muscles since they are most likely to be abnormal—weakness is caused by block of neuromuscular transmission at a proportion of junctions.
- Neuromuscular transmission is enhanced in the cold, so muscles should be warm to maximize any abnormality.
- Usually, in all but the mildest cases, cholinesterase inhibitors do not need to be stopped since neuromuscular transmission remains abnormal despite treatment.

- If testing for myasthenia it is important to study the profile of successive CMAPs in response to a train of stimuli. A decremental response with repetitive stimulation can be seen in a number of settings, including muscles with denervation or **myotonia**. However, the characteristic profile, with minimum CMAP at the fourth or fifth stimulation followed by slight increment, would not be expected in these conditions, nor would the response following brief muscle contraction. Of course abnormalities on routine EMG or other tests should alert the electromyographer to alternative diagnoses.
- SfEMG abnormalities do not always imply the primary site of pathology is the neuromuscular junction. For example, the immature nascent axons and neuromuscular complexes in partially denervated muscle may have variable neuromuscular transmission time. Also watch out for neuromuscular blocking agents in intensive care. Ensure that the clinical presentation fits with neurophysiological findings.

The Role of Neurophysiology in Disorders of Neuromuscular Transmission

Neurophysiological assessment is not always essential in the diagnosis of myasthenia gravis and other disorders of neuromuscular transmission, but a number of studies have reported very high sensitivity and specificity of sfEMG. Provided a weak muscle can be tested, sfEMG is almost invariably abnormal if the pathology lies at the neuromuscular junction (see Table 9.2).

Table 9.2 Sensitivity and specificity of tests of myasthenia gravis. Summary estimate, 95% confidence intervals from clinical trials

	Ocular myasthenia		Generalized myasthenia	
	Sensitivity	**Specificity**	**Sensitivity**	**Specificity**
Tensilon test	0.83–1.00	0.91–1.00	0.78–0.97	0.92–1.00
Antibody to ACh receptor	0.37–0.69	0.95–1.00	0.88–0.99	0.97–1.00
Repetitive nerve stimulation (depends on site and extent of testing)	0.22–0.36	0.91–0.98	0.74–0.84	0.95–0.99
sfEMG orbicularis oculi	0.94–1.00	0.88–0.97		
sfEMG extensor digitorum communis			0.94–1.00	0.95–1.00

Adapted from *Neuromuscular Disorders*, 16 (7), Benatar, M. A systematic review of diagnostic studies in myasthenia gravis, 459, Copyright (2006), with permission from Elsevier.

Or, put the other way, if sfEMG examination of a weak muscle is normal, the cause is almost certainly not myasthenia. Once treatment has been started, sfEMG remains abnormal in all but the mildest cases, so treatment should not be stopped if there is any clinical concern about the safety of doing so. Even localized ocular myasthenia is commonly detected with sfEMG of the orbicularis oculi muscle in patients in whom treatment has been started.

In some settings, particularly research studies, follow-up neurophysiological assessment can be helpful in established myasthenics, but in routine practice treatment is titrated according to symptoms. One special situation is the known myasthenic admitted with an acute deterioration in whom it is not clear whether the presentation is a myasthenic crisis or some other cause of weakness. Severely abnormal repetitive stimulation, and sfEMG if needed, would favour undertreatment, and therefore the diagnosis of a myasthenic crisis.

Chapter 10

Neurophysiology in Clinical Context

Key points

- Some neurophysiological findings may be considered 'hard', reliable predictors of pathology, whereas 'soft', less reliable, findings may be best ignored if they do not fit the clinical context.
- Although some nerve conduction findings are more reliable than others, the magnitude of the abnormality, experience of the examiner, and patient factors, such as oedema, will affect them. Discuss results with the electrophysiologist, especially if they are at odds with clinical expectation.
- An abnormal electrophysiological result that does not fit with expectation may mean your working diagnosis is incorrect. However, it may be a false positive, or a true, but clinically irrelevant, positive.
- If sensory conduction studies are normal despite clear sensory symptoms or signs consider whether proximal pathology is likely.
- Normal motor conduction to a weak muscle raises the possibility of proximal motor conduction block, although there is a wide differential.
- EMG of a weak muscle will reveal essentially normal motor unit action potentials provided there is no motor axon loss and no pathology affecting type I muscle fibres. There are usually other EMG and clinical clues to the diagnosis, including presence of spontaneous activity and the recruitment pattern of motor units.

This chapter could be called 'when to ignore the neurophysiology', because the bottom line with any test result is that it must make sense given the clinical context, and if not it should be treated with suspicion and may be best ignored. However, there are a number of settings in which neurophysiological findings might not match expectation, and familiarity with these scenarios avoids confusion. When any unexpected test result is obtained, the first step should be to retake the history and re-examine the patient to double check the clinical presentation. If the neurophysiology still makes no sense it may be best to discount it, but this should only be done after proper consideration.

There are two common scenarios, addressed in turn in the rest of this chapter:

1. An abnormality is found on neurophysiological examination but it doesn't explain or fit the clinical presentation.
2. The neurophysiological examination is normal despite a clear clinical deficit.

The process of assessing test results and determining their significance in light of the clinical presentation is typically the responsibility of the electrodiagnostic physician who examined the patient and performed the test. It is this judgement, and clinical opinion, which requires a physician to interpret these tests. However, with increasing reliance on technician-led nerve conduction clinics and result reporting, this role is increasingly transferred to the requesting physician. They of course know the clinical presentation, but may be uncomfortable about determining the significance of neurophysiological test results.

Scenario 1

Ignoring abnormal neurophysiology: hard and soft findings

On some occasions, abnormal neurophysiological findings are best ignored if they do not match those expected from the clinical presentation. However, consideration should be given to how robust the neurophysiological findings are (Table 10.1). The process is analogous to the experienced clinician discounting unreliable findings from the neurological examination. '*Hard*' signs are those that are trusted to reliably indicate pathology, such as failure of abduction of one eye, an extensor plantar response, or absent deep tendon reflex. These contrast with '*soft*' signs, such as mild muscle weakness in the context of pain, or an ill-defined patch of altered skin sensation, which are less robust indicators of pathology. When interpreting results, the hard signs are given more weight than the softer findings, some of which can be discounted. Understanding how to weight examination findings is a fundamental part of becoming an experienced neurologist—knowing what to ignore—yet it is impossible to agree on a table of hard and soft signs since it depends on clinical context. Exactly the same is true in clinical neurophysiology (which is often said to be 'an extension of the neurological examination')—hard and

Table 10.1 How robust are the neurophysiological results? Several factors need to be considered to determine the likely reliability and reproducibility of results

Results	Is the nerve commonly and easily recorded? (see also Table 10.2) What is the magnitude of the abnormality? What is the amplitude and duration of the response? • Low amplitude: mild conduction slowing does not imply demyelination • Long duration: apparent conduction block may in fact be temporal dispersion Is the abnormality isolated or are there other corresponding abnormalities? Does EMG fit with nerve conduction results?
Patient	Could results be explained by a common anatomical variant? Are there relevant patient factors: oedema, obesity, cooperation, cold extremities?
Examiner	What is the experience of the examiner, both in performing the test and interpreting the result?
Overall	Does the abnormality make sense given the clinical presentation?

soft findings must be understood, but are almost impossible to list in a table because it lacks context.

In the neurophysiological examination, examples of 'hard' findings include fibrillation potentials on EMG, or severely abnormal conduction studies from a nerve that is generally easily and reliably recorded, such as forearm median motor conduction. 'Soft' neurophysiological findings can include mildly abnormal nerve conduction studies of unusual or difficult to record nerves, particularly small sensory nerves, or an isolated reduction in the interference pattern on EMG without convincing abnormality of the motor unit action potentials. This, of course, is where clinical context and the experience of the examiner are crucial. Do not unquestioningly accept the tables of numbers in a neurophysiological report—some are more reliable and reproducible than others. For example, the test–retest variability is much higher for sensory response amplitudes (SNAP amplitudes) than for motor conduction velocities.

Table 10.2 is provided as a very rough guide to introduce the concept of reliability of common neurophysiological findings. It is of course flawed and can never substitute for discussing the case with the physician who performed the test. Although some tests are inherently rather less reliable than others, there are a host of other factors that need to be considered including the magnitude of abnormality, the examiner's experience and various patient factors. If a test is performed poorly, or there is a source of interference, it is far more likely that abnormal results are recorded from a normal nerve or muscle than vice versa.

Table 10.2 A rough guide to stimulate consideration of the reliability of common neurophysiological findings (number of ticks corresponds roughly to reliability/reproducibility). Of course reliability depends on many factors including the magnitude of the abnormality and the experience of the examining physician. In general, less commonly examined nerves should be considered less reliable. Note that the table is no substitute for discussing the case with the physician who performed the examination.

(a) Motor nerves

	Distal latency	Amplitude	Conduction velocity	Comment
Median	✓✓✓	✓✓✓	✓✓✓	Stimulation above the elbow may also excite the ulnar nerve to thenar muscles, potentially confounding results when there is a severe neuropathy. Median neuropathy at the wrist is a common incidental finding
Ulnar	✓✓✓	✓✓✓	✓✓✓	Conduction velocity around the elbow can be affected by inaccurate measurement of distance, and by temperature
Radial	✓✓	✓✓	✓✓	Relatively hard to locate sites for stimulation proximal to the forearm, and CMAP may be affected by coactivation of nearby muscles
Tibial	✓✓	✓✓	✓✓	Proximal stimulation at the knee is commonly submaximal, so diagnosis of conduction block may be doubtful. Cold feet causes prolonged **distal latency**
Deep peroneal	✓	✓	✓✓	The extensor digitorum brevis muscle may be asymmetrically atrophied in normal people, for example, due to repeated minor trauma

Median nerve conduction to abductor pollicis brevis, ulnar to abductor digiti minimi, radial to extensor indicis proprius, tibial to abductor hallucis, deep peroneal to extensor digitorum brevis.

Table 10.2 (Continued)

(b) Sensory nerves

	Amplitude	Conduction velocity	Comment
Median	✓✓	✓✓	Median neuropathy at the wrist is a common incidental finding. Cold hands reduce conduction velocity
Ulnar	✓✓	✓✓	Conduction velocity reduced by cold. Amplitude may be reduced in adults whose hands are calloused from strenuous manual work
Radial	✓✓	✓✓	The last sensory nerve to be lost with progression of a length dependent peripheral neuropathy. Rarely affected by entrapment
Sural	✓✓	✓	Often unobtainable if there is ankle oedema. Absence not necessarily pathological if >70 years old. Cold affects conduction velocity
Superficial peroneal	✓	✓	May be lost due to minor trauma, so absence not necessarily pathological depending on context, age

(c) EMG

	Overall reliability	Comment
EMG	✓✓ to ✓✓✓	The finding of fibrillation potentials is robust. Minor abnormalities of motor unit action potential morphology or interference pattern are less reliable in isolation. Robust results are obtained when a thorough examination is performed by an experienced operator and the EMG parameters correspond to one another

The risk, therefore, is that a diagnosis is made on the basis of a false positive result, which is why a neurophysiological test result that does not fit with clinical expectation should be treated with suspicion. Of course, the numerous individual test results that make up a complete neurophysiological examination do not stand in isolation, and there is usually internal consistency of findings, meaning that significant pathologies are often detected by at least two individual test parameters.

Abnormal test results that do not fit the clinical presentation fall into two categories.

1. *True but irrelevant positives*: sometimes small nerves are damaged for trivial or unknown reasons not related to the clinical presentation, thus although the test reliably indicates an abnormality it is not clinically relevant.
   - The superficial peroneal sensory nerve is easily damaged, for example, by wearing tight-fitting shoes, so its absence is not always indicative of relevant pathology, particularly in more elderly patients.
   - The peroneal nerve motor response from the extensor digitorum brevis can be asymmetrical for unknown reason or due to minor local trauma irrelevant to the clinical context. Thus, recording a small CMAP from the extensor digitorum brevis, or finding EMG evidence of denervation of this muscle, is not necessarily useful.
   - A small ulnar sensory response from the little finger is relatively common in patients with calloused hands who perform a lot of hard manual work, so should be interpreted with caution in this context.
   - Median neuropathy at the wrist is common, but not always associated with symptoms to make the diagnosis of carpal tunnel syndrome. It is frequently mild and not relevant, and should not be treated.
2. *False positives*: the test is abnormal but there is no pathology—the error lies with the neurophysiology. There are a number of reasons why this might occur:
   - *Some nerves are hard to record.* Many small sensory nerves only give rise to low-amplitude responses, which can be hard to detect if their course is variable or there is overlying adipose tissue. The lateral cutaneous nerve of the thigh is a well-known example, and is often unrecordable even on the asymptomatic side in patients with meralgia paraesthetica, so absence of a response is not necessarily pathological. Furthermore, many small sensory nerves are not commonly tested, so the lack of familiarity of the examiner may be a source of error.
   - *In some situations a nerve which usually yields robust results may become less reliable.* Stimulation of the median nerve with recording electrodes over abductor pollicis brevis usually gives robust results, and is very commonly performed. However, if the CMAP is small and the nerve is difficult to excite, for example, in some demyelinating neuropathies, it is easy to get spurious results from proximal stimulation above the elbow. The reason is that in this context the high stimulus intensity required can easily activate axons in both the median and ulnar nerves.

The recording electrode, over the thenar muscles, will detect muscles activated by both median and ulnar stimulation. Whilst in theory the electrophysiologist may be alerted to inadvertent ulnar nerve stimulation by a change in CMAP shape, this is not always detected when the CMAP is small or dispersed. Note that a similar problem does not tend to occur with ulnar nerve studies, recording over the abductor digiti minimi. Even though proximal stimulation may excite axons in other nerves there are only ulnar innervated muscles in the hypothenar eminence. This means it is easier, and generally more robust, to demonstrate proximal motor conduction block in these ulnar axons than median.

- *A combination of factors may reduce reliability.* Radial nerve motor studies, for example recording over the extensor indicis proprius in the forearm, are generally less robust than routine ulnar or median nerve studies for a number of reasons. They are less frequently performed, single radial muscles are harder to isolate for surface recording, and the radial nerve can be relatively hard to locate for proximal stimulation. Thus, in some situations the results should be treated with caution, for example, when CMAPs are small and dispersed and the nerve is hard to stimulate. Under these conditions there is a tendency for high levels of stimulation to excite adjacent muscles and affect the CMAP.

In some situations it may be important to accept certain parameters of a single nerve conduction study as 'hard', whereas other aspects of that same study may be 'soft'. For example, in a very obese patient a median nerve forearm motor conduction velocity of 22m/s is a hard finding, suggesting demyelination. However, in this patient the finding of an abductor pollicis brevis CMAP of 3.2mV with proximal stimulation compared to 5.5mV with distal stimulation may well not provide good evidence of conduction block if there was difficulty obtaining supramaximal stimulation proximally (it should prompt the examining neurophysiologist to re-examine power of that muscle, since it would be weak if there was true block, to perform EMG, and perhaps also consider a median-ulnar anastomosis).

Scenario 2

The neurophysiology is normal but the patient is not

Of course, one obvious reason for a normal neurophysiological examination is that there is no disease of peripheral nerve or muscle. This is almost always apparent from the history and examination, so causes little confusion and will not be considered further here.

More important is to appreciate the limitations of nerve conduction and EMG—the blind spots when real pathology of the peripheral nerves or muscles may not be detected. Thus the patient with burning limbs may have a small-fibre neuropathy which will not be detected without use of specialist tests. Partial lesions of the nerve roots or plexus may also be very difficult to detect, especially if they are demyelinating and therefore lack accompanying evidence of denervation on EMG. These blind spots are predictable, and in most instances the normality of some neurophysiological findings can be overcome by considering the wider clinical context and the overall patterns of neurophysiological abnormality expected in disease (summarized in Tables 6.2 and 6.3 in Chapter 6).

Electrodiagnosis of peripheral nerve and muscle relies on recording electrical responses from functioning nerve axons and muscle fibres, yet many diseases, for example axonal neuropathies, result in loss of function. Nerve conduction studies, and to some extent EMG too, reflect the remaining functioning fibres—those least affected by disease! Given this, it is not surprising that mild disease resulting in loss of function may pass undetected.

On the other hand, one might expect that a disease process which causes gain of function/abnormality, at least from an electrical perspective, would be more sensitively detected provided the resulting electrical changes stand out from normality. Examples are fibrillation potentials or myotonic discharges on EMG, both of which are sensitively detected.

Sensory symptoms but normal sensory conduction studies

The sensory action potential is a test of the integrity of large-diameter sensory axons in the periphery. It tells us if axonal (but not demyelinating) pathology is pre- or postganglionic since the response amplitude will only be reduced with lesions of large sensory axons at, or distal to, their cell bodies in the dorsal root ganglion. If the pathological process affects only the sensory axon proximal to the dorsal root ganglion there is no Wallerian degeneration of the distal nerve from which the sensory response is recorded. In this, and other scenarios, the distally recorded **sensory potential** will be normal but the patient will have altered sensation.

Normal sensory conduction in a patient with altered sensation

1. Pathology, either axonal or demyelinating, proximal to the dorsal root ganglion ('preganglionic'). This includes the proximal section of the dorsal root as well as central sensory pathways.

2. Conduction block proximal to both the stimulating and recording electrodes, even if the site of block is distal to the dorsal root ganglion. Because there is no axon loss the sensory amplitude is normal. It will only be reduced if the site of block lies between the stimulating and recording electrodes.
3. Acute axonal pathology proximal to the recording and **stimulating electrodes** (same site as (2)) since it takes time for Wallerian degeneration (see Chapter 8).
4. Pathology restricted to small-diameter sensory axons that do not contribute to the sensory nerve action potential, but may still cause burning or pain.
5. Mild pathology sufficient to cause symptoms, but not enough to reduce nerve conduction parameters below the lower limit of the normal range.
6. In theory there could be very distal pathology, beyond both the stimulating and recording electrodes.
7. Functional disease, without organic pathology.

Weakness with normal motor conduction studies

There are many causes of a reduced amplitude CMAP, considered in Chapters 2 and 3. To record a CMAP within the normal range, the distal motor nerve, neuromuscular junction, and to some extent the muscle must all be functioning relatively well. Weakness may of course result from an upper motor neuron lesion, pain, or it could be functional, but these are generally apparent from the clinical presentation and will not be given further consideration here.

There are a number of peripheral neuromuscular disorders to consider, in which weakness is accompanied by normal motor conduction studies. In this setting there are few causes of severe weakness, but milder weakness may be accompanied by a subtle reduction in CMAP which may pass undetected since the amplitude remains within the normal range for the population. In this case needle EMG examination improves the sensitivity of diagnosis.

Normal motor conduction to a *very* weak muscle

1. Motor conduction block proximal to the stimulating electrode. Sometimes proximal nerve root stimulation may demonstrate the block, but this is not always practical. Without axon loss there is no reduction in CMAP amplitude.
2. Acute motor axon loss proximal to the stimulating electrode, tested within a few days of injury. In this case there will not have been time for Wallerian degeneration and reduction in the CMAP. If the lesion lies between the stimulating and recording electrodes it results in a conduction block pattern of results for up to a few days—discussed in Chapter 8.

3. Upper motor neuron pathology, pain, or functional weakness, all generally clinically distinct from peripheral neuromuscular disease.

Normal motor conduction to a *mildly* weak muscle (the small decrease in CMAP amplitude is not detected)

1. Most patients with disease of the neuromuscular junction. Although routine motor conduction may be normal, repetitive stimulation and sfEMG will detect the abnormality. Unlike in myasthenia gravis, the resting CMAP is usually reduced in Lambert–Eaton myasthenic syndrome (Chapter 9).
2. Most patients with myopathy, although the CMAP is reduced in severe disease.
3. Early anterior horn cell disease, before severe muscle wasting.
4. Single level radiculopathies. Since most muscles receive innervation via multiple roots, some remain unaffected, and the CMAP is commonly minimally affected (especially with upper cervical or lumbar radiculopathies).
5. Partial plexopathies. Motor conduction may well remain near normal unless there is quite severe axon loss, particularly with pathology of the upper brachial or lumbar plexus, which are generally less well examined by nerve conduction studies. EMG abnormalities are usually present.

Weakness with normal motor unit action potentials on EMG

It is interesting to consider situations in which motor unit action potential morphology remains normal despite peripheral neuromuscular disease, since it implies there has been insufficient drive, or time, for motor unit remodelling. However, it is important to emphasize that there are often changes in other EMG parameters, such as spontaneous activity or recruitment pattern, which indicate the likely diagnosis (for an overview the reader is referred to Chapters 5 and 6).

Recall that motor unit action potentials that have a long duration, high amplitude, and are polyphasic are sometimes (inaccurately) referred to as 'neurogenic' because they are frequently the result of disease of the anterior horn cell or its axon. They are, however, occasionally also seen with primary muscle pathology. On the other hand, muscle disease or, rarely, severe disease of the neuromuscular junction, will cause 'myopathic' looking motor unit action potentials which are generally low amplitude, short duration, and polyphasic. Similar motor unit action potentials can also result from axon loss/regeneration.

Normal motor unit action potentials from a weak muscle

1. Pure motor conduction block without axon loss. There is no motor unit remodelling, so the motor unit action potentials are normal. However, EMG shows the recruitment of motor units is abnormally reduced, and those units recruited fire at very high rates due to intact central drive.
2. Acute axon loss, before there has been time for motor unit remodelling (a few weeks). But other EMG abnormalities of motor unit recruitment are immediately apparent, and fibrillation potentials develop within 1–3 weeks.
3. Mild disease of the neuromuscular junction. With mild disease the instability of motor unit action potentials may pass unnoticed on routine EMG, and there will be insufficient block to cause motor unit action potentials to be low amplitude and polyphasic (only occurs in severe disease). sfEMG detects the abnormality.
4. Myopathies that only affect type II muscle fibres, such as can occur with steroids, or in muscle wasting associated with chronic disease. The EMG examination primarily studies type I muscle fibres.
5. Upper motor neuron pathology, pain or functional disease—usually clinically apparent.

Chapter 11

Statistics and Neurophysiology

Key points

- For statistical discussion the neurophysiological examination is considered a test, but it is more complex as it involves judgement and a considered clinical opinion in light of the results.
- The ability of the neurophysiologist to confirm or refute a diagnosis depends on the referring clinician since their threshold for referral determines the pre-test odds of disease.
- To confirm a diagnosis requires a positive result from a specific test performed when there is a reasonably high clinical suspicion of that disease.
- Tests can be combined in series provided each is independent from the other, in which case the odds of disease are modified with each test result in turn.
- For longitudinal assessment of a known disease over time the neurophysiological examination need not provide specific results, but they must be reproducible, and sensitive to change.
- To avoid mistakes it is more critical that a neurophysiologist has a good understanding of neurology (or indeed, vice versa) than technical knowledge about how to perform unusual nerve conduction studies.

The Outcome of Testing is Dependent on the Referral

Clinicians generally diagnose by developing a level of suspicion of a disease from the clinical presentation, which can be expressed as the pre-test odds or probability of that disease, then using a test to modify that suspicion, generating post-test odds (Fig. 11.1). Mathematically this was appreciated by Thomas Bayes, and can be expressed as:

Pre-test odds of disease × likelihood ratio from the test = post-test odds

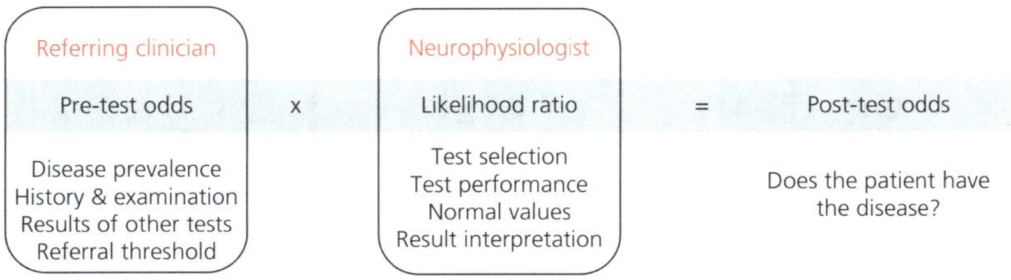

Figure 11.1 The post-test odds that a patient has a disease are determined by the referring clinician and the neurophysiologist.

So the odds that our patient has the disease in question, in other words the post-test odds, will depend on two things:

1. *Likelihood ratio*, which in general is an intrinsic feature of a test, derived from the sensitivity and specificity (see 'Appendix') which we can do little to alter without developing new and better tests. However, the neurophysiological examination, considered as a whole, is rather different because it consists of a combination of tests with clinical opinion. The *electrophysiologist* performing the examination effectively alters the overall likelihood ratio by their experience in the choice and performance of tests, and interpretation of results (considered further later). There are many factors considered, including degree of abnormality, patient habitus, and reliability of results.
2. *Pre-test odds* of disease are determined by an understanding of disease prevalence in the relevant community together with the results of clinical history and examination, and any previous tests. The overall pre-test odds are therefore determined by the threshold at which the *referring clinician* asks for a neurophysiological opinion having assessed the clinical presentation .

The neurophysiologist can only go so far to maximize the likelihood ratio. Thus the outcome and perceived usefulness of a test (here, the neurophysiological examination) will depend to a large extent on the referring clinician's determination of pre-test odds of the disease, according to their referral habits.

Demonstration of the Effect of Pre-test Odds

After tests have been performed, we want to know the chance that the patient has the disease under suspicion—in Bayesian terminology, the post-test odds of disease. In fact, most clinicians are more used to dealing with probabilities of disease than odds, and to thinking in terms of positive predictive values from a test, which tell us the chance that the patient really has a disease if the test comes back positive. For this reason, in the examples given, we will look at the effect of disease prevalence on predictive value of a test (high disease prevalence equating to high pre-test odds of disease). For readers requiring a reminder, the 'Appendix' revises the derivation of probabilities from odds, positive predictive values, likelihood ratios, sensitivities, specificities, and so on.

Let us suppose we have a test with 95% specificity and 85% sensitivity. We have been asked to try and confirm a diagnosis, but the prevalence of disease is 5%, so 500 of 10,000 people will have the disease (Table 11.1):

Table 11.1 Diagnostic testing with 5% disease prevalence (low pre-test odds of disease)

		Target disease		
		Present	**Absent**	
Test result	+	425	475	Positive predictive value 47%
	–	75	9025	Negative predictive value 99%
		Sensitivity 85%	Specificity 95%	

It is clear that with such a low prevalence of disease, even a positive test is unable to confirm the diagnosis: the positive predictive value is poor since the post-test odds of disease remain low. Note, however, that the negative predictive value is high, meaning that a negative result provides strong reassurance that the patient is unaffected. This example shows why the neurophysiological examination may not provide convincing evidence of a disease if the clinical suspicion is low to start with.

Now let us take the same test and imagine that the prevalence of disease is 80%, so 8000 of 10,000 people will have the disease (high pre-test odds of disease) (Table 11.2):

Table 11.2 Diagnostic testing with 80% disease prevalence (high pre-test odds of disease)

		Target disease		
		Present	**Absent**	
Test result	+	6800	100	Positive predictive value 99%
	–	1200	1900	Negative predictive value 61%
		Sensitivity 85%	Specificity 95%	

In this instance a positive test result provides strong support that the patient does indeed have the disease since there are high post-test odds of disease. On the other hand a negative test does little to reassure us that the patient is unaffected when the pre-test odds are so high.

In these examples it is apparent that the pre-test odds of disease will determine whether the test is able to confirm or refute a diagnosis.

- To rule a diagnosis *in* requires a positive result from a specific test performed when there is a high clinical suspicion of that disease.
- To rule a diagnosis *out* requires a negative result from a sensitive test performed when there is a low clinical suspicion of disease.

In the context of the neurophysiological examination it is important to stress that the ability of the neurophysiologist to confirm or refute a diagnosis will depend on whether there is a high or low level of suspicion of that diagnosis.

Get Out What You Put In

It is a statistical inevitability that the output from a clinical neurophysiology department depends on what you put in, which in turn depends on where you work and what type of medicine you practice. Some clinicians request few investigations, and reserve them only for patients in whom they are very suspicious of an abnormality. In this situation the pre-test odds of disease are high, thus a positive test is likely to help give a fairly definite answer. Of course, this physician will make a few type II errors, that is, they will miss a few true cases because of their limited investigation, either through choice or lack or resources.

The alternative approach is to perform lots of tests even though the pre-test odds of disease are relatively low. In this situation, common in tertiary referral centres, the neurophysiological assessment may well be normal or marginally abnormal, which, combined with the low pre-test probability of disease, results in unhelpfully low post-test odds of disease (the clinical neurophysiology department might seem less useful in this setting, 'the results are always normal or uncertain'). The statistical cost of multiple investigations is the higher number of false positives, which both the neurophysiologist and referring clinician need to be aware of in order to minimize type I errors—diagnosing unaffected people with disease.

Multiple Tests

One way in which diagnostic testing can be made more powerful is by combining a number of different tests. Statistically, tests can be combined in series provided each is independent from the other, in which case the odds of disease are modified with each test result in series in a Bayesian manner. Great caution must be exercised, however, since tests are often not fully independent from each other. Furthermore, the false positive rate is cumulative if a single abnormality is accepted as diagnostic; for example, consider how often a single unexpected minor outlier on 'routine' blood screen is dismissed. For this reason it is common to rely on internal consistency of neurophysiological results, that is, more than one abnormal test result indicating the same pathology, before conclusions are drawn. Furthermore, and most importantly, the neurophysiological conclusion of course has to make sense in the wider clinical context.

One attraction of performing multiple independent tests is that, provided they are appropriately interpreted, an accurate diagnosis may be reached despite each individual subtest being rather inaccurate. For example, an expertly interpreted clinical history and examination can often correctly diagnose rare diseases by combining answers to a number of sequential questions, or observations, each of which individually have rather low likelihood ratios. The values of the individual likelihood ratios are often unknown, as in nerve conduction and EMG, but consistency between a number of different strands of evidence gives confidence that the conclusions are correct. To some extent this is what experience and 'getting a feel' for clinical medicine is all about—understanding how to combine and weight evidence to build up a reliable diagnosis. This applies to the neurophysiological examination just as it does the clinical examination. From the perspective of clinical history taking and examination it has been suggested that the minimum useful positive likelihood ratio for each test is about 2, and negative likelihood ratio 0.5, reflecting a relatively inaccurate sensitivity and specificity of about 0.65.

Degree of Abnormality

It is intuitively obvious that the magnitude of abnormality plays a critical role in determining whether the result of a test is trusted, and thus whether a confident diagnosis is made. In statistical terms this is sometimes expressed as multilevel likelihood ratios. For example, a very abnormal result from a robust test, such as median nerve forearm motor conduction velocity of 23m/s, provides a high likelihood ratio, whereas a value that is only slightly abnormal, say 46m/s, produces a much lower likelihood ratio, and has a greater chance of being a false positive, especially if it is unexpected (in other words when the pre-test odds of disease are low).

Changing the Normal Values

When there are low pre-test odds of disease there is a high risk of false positive results from any diagnostic test. The neurophysiologist can reduce the number of false positives simply by increasing the threshold for calling a result abnormal. This widening of the normal range, such that more tests are called normal, increases the specificity whilst reducing the sensitivity of the test. This may be performed intuitively by the neurophysiologist in the final interpretation of the test, and is one of a number of safety mechanisms for not making a potentially devastating diagnosis on the basis of a mildly abnormal test result if the context is not right.

Occasionally, the neurophysiologist might be asked to exclude a diagnosis. To do this requires a negative result from a very sensitive test. The sensitivity of a test will be increased by narrowing the normal range, such that more tests are called abnormal, and by combining a series of tests. Although there will be more false positives, if the result is negative despite these measures the subject is more unlikely to have the disease.

Changing normal values is not generally accepted practice, but is often performed subconsciously in the final interpretation of results. It is not possible to perform nerve conduction and EMG blind to the suspected diagnosis since the clinical presentation determines the nerves and muscles that are tested. Adequate discussion about difficult or atypical examinations and their interpretation is essential. To avoid mistakes it is more critical that an electrophysiologist has a good understanding of the clinical context, that is, the presentation and differential diagnosis (which includes a good referral question), than technical knowledge about how to perform unusual nerve conduction studies.

The Reality of Unknown Statistics in Clinical Neurophysiology

In order to practise evidence-based medicine a diagnostic test, neurophysiological or otherwise, should be assessed against a gold standard. However, there are a number of problems in determining the precise likelihood ratio or positive predictive value of many neurophysiological tests. Perhaps most difficult to overcome is the fact that there is often no gold standard with which to compare the test result. If nerve conduction and EMG is one of the primary methods of establishing the diagnosis and quantifying disease, for example, in large-fibre neuropathies, the test will be accurate by definition!

Another major hurdle is that the neurophysiological examination is operator dependent, with variation in the type and number of tests chosen, how technically well they are performed and how they are interpreted. Furthermore, normal ranges vary between different labs. In the ideal world there would be standardization of testing, but this is not the case. Although some general rules apply, it is up to each electrophysiologist to understand the normal ranges of the lab in which they work, and determine which tests give high likelihood ratios in their hands.

These difficulties should not stop attempts to quantify likelihood ratios and validate neurophysiological techniques. However, in the meantime it is true to say that, although not always backed by precise quantitative evidence, the neurophysiological examination remains helpful and valid—just like the clinical history and examination.

Select Reproducible Tests for Longitudinal Assessment

Nerve conduction and EMG are usually used for diagnosis, but sometimes patients with a known diagnosis are referred in order to provide objective evidence about change in disease over time. One example would be the use of sensory and motor response amplitudes to track changes in an axonal neuropathy. In this situation it is not necessary to perform a very specific examination, such as might be appropriate for diagnosis, but ideally the testing should be:

1. Sensitive, to detect minor changes.
2. Reproducible when re-measured.
3. Able to capture progression of pathology. In other words, the test parameters must change as the disease progresses, and not miss relevant change.

Provided these conditions are met, and the diagnosis is not in question, then a limited number of neurophysiological tests may be useful as measures of disease progression and treatment efficacy. An analogy might be the use of the erythrocyte sedimentation rate to follow progression of some inflammatory conditions; it is sensitive to change but not specific to that condition. Of course, should the diagnosis be called into question the neurophysiological approach needs to be modified to reflect this, with greater emphasis on specific tests.

From the neurophysiological examination some parameters are more reproducible with retesting than others, for example, sensory and motor response amplitudes may vary by as much as 50% with repetition, although good technique will limit this. In comparison, conduction velocity and minimum F-wave latency vary by less than 20%.

Further reading

Gill CJ, Sabin L, Schmid CH. Why clinicians are natural Bayesians. *Br Med J* 2005; **330**: 1080–3.

Straus SE, Richardson WS, Glasziou P, Haynes RB. *Evidence based medicine. How to practice and teach EBM*, 3rd edition. Elsevier: Edinburgh, 2005.

Appendix

In order to assess the accuracy of a test it is performed on a population, and compared against a gold standard (Table 11.3).

Table 11.3 Assessment of test accuracy in a population with the target disorder

Test result	Target disorder		
	Present	**Absent**	
+	a	b	Positive predictive value a/(a+b)
–	c	d	Negative predictive value d/(c+d)
	Sensitivity a/(a+c)	Specificity d/(b+d)	

Prevalence = (a+c)/(a+b+c+d)

Pre-test odds = prevalence/(1 – prevalence)

Positive likelihood ratio (LR+) = sensitivity/(1 – specificity)

Negative likelihood ratio (LR-) = (1 – sensitivity)/specificity

Post-test odds = pre-test odds × likelihood ratio

Post-test probability = post-test odds/(post-test odds +1)

Section 2

Chapter 12

Reference

Differential Diagnoses

The differential diagnoses are arranged assuming that both the clinical presentation and results of nerve conduction and EMG are known. Thus, for example, the presence or absence of demyelination is known. The aim is to help clinicians recall differential diagnoses that integrate clinical presentation with electrodiagnostic results.

Generalized or widespread presentations

Axonal sensorimotor peripheral neuropathies

Acute/subacute

- Acute motor and sensory axonal neuropathy (AMSAN) variant of Guillain–Barré syndrome
- Critical illness neuropathy
- Porphyria
- Graft-versus-host disease
- Tick paralysis (nerve or neuromuscular junction)
- *Toxic*: some drugs (see 'Chronic/subacute'), lead, mercury, arsenic, thallium.

Chronic/subacute

- *Metabolic/nutritional*: diabetes, vitamin B12, uraemia, hepatic failure, hypothyroid, folate, thiamine, vitamin E, copper, acromegaly, after bariatric surgery
- *Infectious*: HIV, Lyme disease, hepatitis C, HTLV-1, Whipple's disease

Axonal sensorimotor peripheral neuropathies *(Continued)*

- *Hereditary*: Charcot–Marie–Tooth type 2, glycogen storage disease, acanthocytosis syndromes, abetalipoproteinaemia, cerebrotendinous xanthomatosis
- *Medication/toxic*: vincristine, cisplatin, paclitaxel, nitrofurantoin, chloramphenicol, pyridoxine, thalidomide, phenytoin, isoniazid, hydralazine, amiodarone, alcohol
- *Other inflammatory*: Sjögren's syndrome, systemic lupus erythematosus, rheumatoid arthritis, coeliac, sarcoidosis, scleroderma, primary biliary cirrhosis, graft-versus-host disease
- *Paraprotein*: MGUS (IgG/IgA), amyloid, Waldenström's macroglobulinaemia, cryoglobulinaemia
- *Paraneoplastic*: several, often with ataxia and other signs
- *Neoplastic infiltration*: leukaemia, lymphoma, multiple myeloma, neurofibromatosis
- Idiopathic

HTLV-1, human T-cell lymphotrophic virus type 1; Ig, immunoglobulin; MGUS, monoclonal gammopathy of uncertain significance.

Demyelinating peripheral neuropathies

Acute/subacute

- Guillain–Barré syndrome
- *Toxic/medication*: amiodarone, tacrolimus, antibodies to TNF-α, bortezomib, perhexilene, cytosine arabinoside, arsenic, n-hexane
- Graft-versus-host disease
- Diphtheria neuropathy

Chronic/subacute

- *Chronic inflammatory demyelinating neuropathy:* may be associated with HIV, diabetes, hepatitis B and C, systemic lupus erythematosus, inflammatory bowel disease
- Multifocal motor neuropathy with conduction block

Demyelinating peripheral neuropathies *(Continued)*

- Pure motor demyelinating neuropathy
- *Neuropathies associated with lymphoproliferative diseases/paraproteins*: MGUS (IgM/anti-MAG, IgG, IgA) osteosclerotic myeloma, POEMS, GALOP syndrome, Waldenström's macroglobulinaemia, Castleman disease, lymphoma
- *Charcot–Marie–Tooth disease:* type 1, 3 (Dejerine–Sottas disease), 4, X-linked and dominant-intermediate forms. Also hereditary neuropathy with liability to pressure palsies
- *Other rare genetic conditions*: adrenoleucodystrophy, metachromatic leucodystrophy, adrenomyeloneuropathy, Krabbe's disease, Refsum's disease, Tangier disease, familial amyloid polyneuropathy with transthyretin mutation, cerebrotendinous xanthomatosis, rarely neurofibromatosis 1 and 2, MNGIE.

Ig, immunoglobulin; MAG, myelin associated glycoprotein; GALOP syndrome, gait disorder, autoantibody, late-age onset, polyneuropathy; MGUS, monoclonal gammopathy of uncertain significance; POEMS, polyneuropathy, organomegaly, endocrinopathy, M-band in serum and skin changes; MNGIE, a mitochondrial disease with myopathy and external ophthalmoplegia, neuropathy, gastro-intestinal features, encephalopathy.

Mononeuritis multiplex

Axonal

- *Vasculitis:* polyarteritis nodosa, granulomatosis with polyangiitis (Wegener's), Churg–Strauss, microscopic polyangiitis, Behçet's disease, drug or infection induced, related to systemic lupus erythematosus or rheumatoid arthritis, paraneoplastic vasculitis only affecting peripheral nerves
- *Infection*: HIV, Lyme disease, cytomegalovirus, hepatitis C or B, leprosy
- Sarcoidosis
- Infiltration e.g. lymphoma, or compression e.g. schwannoma
- Vascular occlusion: cholesterol emboli, sickle cell disease
- Diabetes (rare)

Mononeuritis multiplex *(Continued)*

- Multifocal acquired motor axonopathy (motor only)
- Wartenberg's migratory sensory neuritis (sensory only).

Demyelinating

- Multiple entrapments, consider hereditary neuropathy with liability to pressure palsies, amyloidosis, diabetes
- Some variants of chronic inflammatory demyelinating neuropathy (MADSAM)
- Rarely hereditary demyelinating neuropathies: X-linked CMT
- Rarely Guillain–Barré syndrome
- Multifocal motor neuropathy with conduction block (motor only).

MADSAM, multifocal acquired demyelinating sensory and motor neuropathy. CMT, Charcot-Marie-Tooth disease

Ataxic sensory neuropathies/neuronopathies

Sensory neuronopathy/ganglionopathy

- *Paraneoplastic* (anti-Hu): small cell lung cancer commonest, also lung adenocarcinoma, breast, ovarian, lymphoma
- *Inflammatory*: Sjögren's syndrome commonest, rheumatoid arthritis, systemic lupus erythematosus, autoimmune hepatitis
- *Infections*: HIV, Epstein–Barr virus, Lyme, HTLV-1, VZV
- *Toxic/medication*: platinum-based chemotherapy (cisplatin, oxaliplatin), thalidomide, linezolid, taxanes, metronidazole, pyridoxine (vitamin B6) excess
- *Deficiency*: B12, copper
- Idiopathic
- Tabes dorsalis (prominent dorsal column involvement, but dorsal horn involved too)
- *Hereditary*: spinocerebellar ataxias, Friedreich's ataxia, ataxic mitochondrial neuropathies (MIRAS, NARP).

Ataxic sensory neuropathies/neuronopathies *(Continued)*

Demyelination

- Miller Fisher variant of Guillain–Barré syndrome
- Sensory CIDP/AIDP variants, some with dorsal root ganglion involvement
- Monoclonal gammopathy of uncertain significance with IgM/anti-MAG
- Chronic ataxic neuropathy with ophthalmoplegia (CANOMAD)
- Neuropathy with anti-sulfatide antibodies.

CANOMAD, chronic ataxic neuropathy, ophthalmoplegia, IgM paraprotein, cold agglutinin and disialosyl antibodies; HTLV-1 human T-cell lymphotrophic virus type 1; CIDP, chronic inflammatory demyelinating polyneuropathy; AIDP, acute inflammatory demyelinating polyneuropathy; MAG, myelin associated glycoprotein; MIRAS, mitochondrial recessive ataxia syndrome; NARP, neuropathy, ataxia and retinitis pigmentosa; VZV, varicella zoster virus.

Small-fibre sensory neuropathies

- *Diabetic polyneuropathy with small-fibre involvement
- *Amyloid, both familial and acquired
- *Idiopathic
- *HIV neuropathy
- *Alcoholic neuropathy (pain common, autonomic involvement rare)
- **Connective tissue disorders*: Sjögren's syndrome, systemic lupus erythematosus (pain >autonomic involvement)
- Guillain–Barré syndrome
- Fabry's disease, Tangier's.
- Porphyria
- Hereditary sensory and autonomic neuropathies
- Leprosy

* These neuropathies tend to cause prominent pain. Some result in loss of pain sensibility (e.g. hereditary sensory and autonomic neuropathies).

Autonomic neuropathies

- Diabetes
- Amyloid
- Guillain–Barré syndrome
- Paraneoplastic, especially small cell lung cancer
- Idiopathic
- *Infection*: HIV neuropathy, leprosy
- *Multisystem*: multisystem atrophy, mitochondrial
- *Drugs/toxic*: vincristine, taxols, cisplatin, amiodarone, perhexiline, thallium, arsenic, organic solvents, acrylamide
- Hereditary sensory and autonomic neuropathies
- Acute pandysautonomia

Motor predominant peripheral neuropathies/ neuronopathies

- *Asymmetric with upper motor neuron signs:* motor neuron disease, frontotemporal dementia with motor neuron degeneration, AAA syndrome
- *Asymmetric:* multifocal motor neuropathy with conduction block, brachial neuritis, primary muscular atrophy, monomelic amyotrophy, paraneoplastic, polio
- *Symmetric and proximal:* spinal muscular atrophy, bulbo-spinal muscular atrophy (Kennedy's)
- *Acute onset:* Acute motor axonal neuropathy variant of Guillain-Barre Syndrome, porphyria
- *Acquired:* Lead, dapsone, botulism, tick paralysis
- *Distal symmetrical weakness*: Distal spinal muscular atrophies/hereditary motor neuropathies (contrast with distal myopathies)
- *Neuropathies where symptoms are motor >> sensory*: chronic inflammatory demyelinating polyneuropathy, Charcot-Marie-Tooth disease

AAA, achalasia addisonianism alacrima (Allgrove syndrome).
Also consider myasthenia gravis, myopathies in the differential of weakness without sensory loss

Sensorimotor neuronopathy (proximal/cranial presentation)

- *Syringomyelia/syringobulbia
- Bulbospinal muscular atrophy (Kennedy's syndrome)
- Amyloid
- Neurosarcoidosis
- Sjögren's syndrome
- Chronic ataxic neuropathy, ophthalmoplegia, IgM paraprotein, cold agglutinins and disialosyl antibodies (CANOMAD)
- *Facial onset sensory and motor neuronopathy (FOSMN)
- *Tangier disease
- *Lepromatous leprosy.

*Caudal predominant in some. Ig, immunoglobulin.

Polyneuropathy + optic neuropathy

- Copper deficiency
- Friedreich's ataxia
- Leber's hereditary optic neuropathy
- Charcot–Marie–Tooth 2a and 6 (mitofusin 2 mutation)
- *Toxic/drug*: cyanide (from cassava), amiodarone, chloramphenicol, isoniazid, linezolid, vincristine, disulphiram, nitrous oxide, mercury
- Tobacco-alcohol amblyopia.
- Sarcoid (cranial neuropathy rather than peripheral)

Polyneuropathy + myopathy

- Paraneoplastic (mainly sensory neuropathy, type II muscle fibre myopathy)
- *Connective tissue diseases*: systemic lupus erythematosus, rheumatoid arthritis, Sjogren's syndrome, polyarteritis nodosa, mixed connective tissue disease

Polyneuropathy + myopathy *(Continued)*

- Critical illness neuropathy plus myopathy
- Mitochondrial disease
- Inclusion body myositis
- Sarcoidosis
- *Endocrine*: acromegaly, hypothyroid, hyperthyroid
- *Infectious*: Lyme disease, HIV, HTLV-1
- *Toxic/drugs*: alcohol, vincristine, amiodarone, colchicine, chloroquine, doxorubicin, organophosphates, clofibrate
- *Metabolic myopathies*: acid maltase deficiency, debrancher enzyme deficiency.

HTLV-1, human T-cell lymphotrophic virus type 1.

Ascending paralysis, progressing from legs to arms over a few days

- Guillain–Barré syndrome
- Porphyria
- Tick paralysis
- Severe hypophosphataemia
- Diphtheria neuropathy

Distinguish ascending paralysis from the following:

- *Acute generalized flaccid weakness*: myasthenia gravis, intoxication, acute central pathology
- *Acute weakness with respiratory failure*: motor neuron disease, myasthenia gravis, acid maltase deficiency
- *Descending paralysis*: botulism (visual symptoms early, dilated pupils, bulbar involvement then limb weakness)
- *Paralysis developing following prolonged ITU admission*: critical illness neuropathy/myopathy.

Focal clinical presentation

Complex ophthalmoplegia

Acute

- Miller Fisher syndrome
- Botulism
- Tick paralysis
- Brainstem stroke
- Diphtheria

Chronic

- Myasthenia gravis
- Thyroid ophthalmopathy
- Oculopharyngeal muscular dystrophy
- *Mitochondrial*: Progressive external ophthalmoplegia, Kearns–Sayre syndrome
- Congenital myasthenic syndromes
- *Congenital ophthalmoplegias*: centronuclear myopathy, Möbius syndrome, Duane syndrome
- Chronic ataxic neuropathy, ophthalmoplegia, IgM paraprotein, cold agglutinins and disialosyl antibodies (CANOMAD)
- *Mechanical*: masses in orbital fossa, muscle fibrosis.

Bilateral facial palsy

Acute/subacute

- Guillain–Barré syndrome
- Sarcoidosis
- Lyme disease
- Bilateral Bell's palsy
- HIV seroconversion
- Melkersson–Rosenthal syndrome
- Neoplastic infiltration of cranial nerves

Bilateral facial palsy *(Continued)*

Chronic/subacute

- Myasthenia gravis
- Facioscapulohumeral dystrophy
- Myotonic dystrophy
- Bulbospinal muscular atrophy (Kennedy's syndrome)
- Centronuclear and nemaline myopathies
- Möbius syndrome
- Leprosy

Examine for a complex opthalmoplegia to help determine aetiology

Bulbar palsy (dysphonia, dysphagia)

Acute/subacute

- Brainstem stroke
- Guillain–Barré syndrome
- Hypoglossal neuropathy
- *Infection*: botulism, tetanus

Chronic/subacute

- Myasthenia gravis
- Motor neuron disease
- Polymyositis
- Inclusion body myositis
- Bulbospinal muscular atrophy (Kennedy's syndrome)
- Oculopharyngeal muscular dystrophy
- Thyroid disorders
- Myotonic dystrophy
- Syringobulbia
- Allgrove syndrome (Achalasia-Addisonianism-Alacrima)
- Facial onset sensory and motor neuronopathy (FOSMN)

Camptocormia—'dropped head'

- Motor neuron disease
- Myasthenia gravis
- Polymyositis
- Inclusion body myositis
- Local paraspinal myopathy
- Local neck irradiation
- Syringomyelia
- Other hereditary and endocrine myopathies.

Differentiate from dystonic anterocollis where there is tonic spasm of neck muscles, also from extrapyramidal disorders such as Parkinson's disease, and fixed neck flexion with spinal pathology.

Respiratory failure and trunk weakness at presentation

- Motor neuron disease
- Myasthenia gravis
- Adult-onset acid maltase deficiency
- Mitochondrial myopathies
- Muscular dystrophies
- Polymyositis
- Guillain–Barré syndrome
- Brachial neuritis
- Nemaline myopathy

In general, with acute neuromuscular paralysis the neck, shoulder, and diaphragm muscles are roughly equally weak as they share innervation. Respiratory muscle weakness is common at the end stage of many neuromuscular disorders.

Weak finger extension

- Radial neuropathy
- Posterior interosseous neuropathy
- Multifocal motor neuropathy with conduction block
- Posterior cord of brachial plexus (deltoid also weak)
- C7 radiculopathy
- Motor neuron disease.

Not neurogenic

- Rupture of finger extensors (patients with arthritis)
- Rare myopathies: Welander, Gowers (look for more widespread weakness)

Foot drop

Common, unilateral

- Common peroneal neuropathy
- Deep peroneal neuropathy
- Radiculopathy, L4/5
- Motor neuron disease
- Sciatic neuropathy
- Lumbosacral plexopathy
- Compartment syndrome

Bilateral foot drop

- Polyneuropathy, many types
- Cauda equina or conus medullaris lesion
- Bilateral peroneal neuropathies (consider hereditary liability to pressure palsies)
- Distal spinal muscular atrophy/hereditary motor neuropathy
- Scapuloperoneal muscular dystrophy

Foot drop *(Continued)*

- Myotonic dystrophy type 1
- Distal myopathy
- Central, including parasagittal lesions.

Wasting of intrinsic hand muscles

- Ulnar neuropathy (thenar sparing)
- Median neuropathy (only thenar muscles affected)
- Radiculopathy, especially T1
- Lower brachial plexopathy
- Anterior horn cell disease at T1/C8
- Disuse, e.g. severe arthritis
- Severe length dependent neuropathies
- Multifocal motor neuropathy with conduction block (some axon loss and wasting common)
- Distal myopathies (intrinsic hand and foot muscles may be relatively spared)

'Split hand'

- Amyotrophic lateral sclerosis
- Spinal muscular atrophy
- Poliomyelitis
- Charcot–Marie–Tooth 2D (*GARS* mutation)

'Split hand' = wasting of the thenar eminence and 1st dorsal interosseous with relative sparing of the hypothenar eminence. Suggestive of pathology at the level of the anterior horn cell.

Bilateral flail arm (flaccid proximal weakness)

- Motor neuron disease
- Brachial neuritis

Bilateral flail arm (flaccid proximal weakness) *(Continued)*

- Guillain–Barré syndrome
- Cervical cord lesion
- Paraneoplastic neuropathy
- Amyloid neuropathy
- Lyme disease

Flail arms would be a very unusual presentation of primary muscle disease.

Isolated quadriceps femoris weakness

- Disuse atrophy
- Femoral neuropathy
- Diabetic amyotrophy
- L3/4 radiculopathy
- Lumbar plexopathy, especially neoplastic
- Inclusion body myositis
- Muscular dystrophy: Becker, limb girdle
- Focal myositis.

Scapuloperoneal syndromes

Myopathic

- Scapuloperoneal muscular dystrophy
- Facioscapulohumeral dystrophy
- Emery–Dreifuss muscular dystrophy (contractures)
- Limb girdle muscular dystrophy 2A
- Centronuclear myopathy
- *Glycogen storage*: acid maltase deficiency, glycogen phosphorylase deficiency.

Neurogenic

- Davidenkow's syndrome (a neuropathy)
- Scapuloperoneal neuronopathy (a hereditary motor neuronopathy).

See Table 12.1 for clinical presentation of scapular winging.

Table 12.1 Scapular winging. Presentation depends on the weak muscle

	Serratus anterior (long thoracic nerve, C5–7)	Trapezius (spinal accessory nerve, C1–4)	Rhomboids (dorsal scapular nerve, C5)
Degree of winging at rest	Prominent, all of medial (vertebral) border	Minimal, mainly inferior angle displaced laterally and upward	Moderate, displaced laterally
Shoulder position at rest	No true dropping of shoulder	Shoulder is dropped, asymmetric shrug, prominent levator scapulae	No true dropping
Winging exacerbated by	Forward flexion of the arm	Lateral abduction	Lateral abduction causes medial rotation of lower scapular
Winging reduced by	Lateral abduction	Forward flexion	Elevation overhead
Causes	Neuralgic amyotrophy, trauma to chest wall, stretch injury, surgical (1st rib, radical mastectomy), scapuloperoneal syndromes	Procedures in posterior triangle of neck (lymph node biopsy). If the lesion is proximal, also get sternocleidomastoid weakness	Thoracolumbar orthosis bracing for scoliosis, entrapment due to middle scalene hypertrophy

More widespread muscle weakness—see 'Scapuloperoneal syndromes'

Normal values, nerve conduction

See Tables 12.2 and 12.3 for normal values of commonly tested sensory and motor nerves.

Table 12.2 Normal nerve conduction parameters—sensory nerves

Nerve	Stimulation	Recording	Amplitude (μV)	Conduction velocity (m/s)
Median	Index finger	Wrist	≥7	≥49
Ulnar	Little finger	Wrist	≥5	≥49
Radial	Forearm	Snuff box	≥12	≥50
Sural	Calf	Posterior ankle	≥10	≥40
Superficial peroneal	Lateral ankle	Dorsum of foot	≥5	≥40

Table 12.3 Normal nerve conduction parameters—motor nerves

Nerve	Stimulation	Recording	Amplitude (mV)	Onset latency (ms)	Conduction velocity (m/s)	F-wave latency (ms)
Median	Wrist	APB	≥4	≤4.2		≤31
	Elbow	APB			≥49	
Ulnar	Wrist	ADM	≥6	≤3.3		≤32
	Below elbow	ADM			≥49	
Tibial	Ankle	AH	≥4	≤5.8		≤56
	Knee	AH			≥41	
Peroneal	Ankle	EDB	≥2	≤6.5		≤56
	Fibular head	EDB			≥41	

APB, abductor pollicis brevis; ADM, abductor digiti minimi; AH, abductor hallucis brevis; EDB, extensor digitorum brevis.

Note: laboratories use different reference ranges, so check with your local neurophysiologists. You will not be far wrong if you remember normal sensory and motor conduction velocities should be 50m/s in the upper limbs, and 40m/s in the lower limbs. Of course normal values for F-wave latency should be corrected according to height.

Normal nerve root supplies

See Table 12.4 for the nerve and root supply of commonly tested muscles, and Table 12.5 for the root supplies of commonly tested sensory nerves.

Table 12.4 Nerve and root supply of commonly tested muscles. The dominant root is shown in bold.

Upper limb	Spinal roots
Spinal accessory nerve	
Trapezius	XI and C3, C4
Sternocleidomastoid	XI and C2, **C3**, **C4**
Brachial plexus	
Rhomboids (dorsal scapular nerve)	C4, **C5**
Serratus anterior (long thoracic nerve)	C5, C6, C7
Pectoralis major, clavicular head (lateral pectoral nerve)	**C5**, C6
Pectoralis major, sternal head (medial pectoral nerve)	C7, C8, T1

(Continued)

Table 12.4 (Continued)

Upper limb	**Spinal roots**
Supraspinatus (suprascapular nerve)	**C5**, C6
Infraspinatus (suprascapular nerve)	**C5**, C6
Latissimus dorsi (thoracodorsal nerve)	C6, **C7**, C8
Axillary nerve	
Deltoid	**C5**, C6
Musculocutaneous nerve	
Biceps	C5, C6
Radial nerve	
Triceps, lateral, long and medial heads	C6, **C7**, C8
Brachioradialis	C5, **C6**
Extensor carpi radialis longus	C5, **C6**
Posterior interosseous nerve	
Supinator	C6, C7
Extensor carpi ulnaris	**C7**, C8
Extensor digitorum communis	**C7**, C8
Abductor pollicis longus	**C7**, C8
Extensor pollicis longus	**C7**, C8
Extensor pollicis brevis	**C7**, C8
Extensor indicis	**C7**, C8
Median nerve	
Pronator teres	C6, C7
Flexor carpi radialis	C6, C7
Flexor digitorum superficialis	C7, **C8**, T1
Abductor pollicis brevis	C8, **T1**
Flexor pollicis brevis (may be supplied by the ulnar nerve)	C8, **T1**
Opponens pollicis	C8, **T1**
Lumbricals I & II	C8, **T1**
Anterior interosseous nerve	
Flexor digitorum profundus I & II	C7, **C8**
Flexor pollicis longus	C7, **C8**
Ulnar nerve	
Flexor carpi ulnaris	C7, **C8**, T1

(Continued)

Table 12.4 (Continued)

Upper limb	Spinal roots
Flexor digitorum profundus III & IV	C7, **C8**
Hypothenar muscles	C8, **T1**
Adductor pollicis	C8, **T1**
Flexor pollicis brevis	C8, **T1**
Palmar interossei	C8, **T1**
Dorsal interossei	C8, **T1**
Lumbricals III & IV	C8, **T1**
Lower limb	
Femoral nerve	
Iliopsoas	L1, **L2**, L3
Rectus femoris	L2, **L3, L4**
Vastus lateralis, intermedius and medialis	L2, **L3, L4**
Obturator nerve	
Adductor longus	L2, L3, L4
Adductor magnus	L2, L3, L4
Superior gluteal nerve	
Gluteus medius and minimus	**L4, L5**, S1
Tensor fasciae latae	**L4, L5**, S1
Inferior gluteal nerve	
Gluteus maximus	**L5, S1**, S2
Sciatic and tibial nerves	
Semitendinosus	L5, **S1**, S2
Semimembranosus	L5, **S1**, S2
Biceps femoris	L5, **S1**, S2
Gastrocnemius and soleus	S1, S2
Tibialis posterior	L4, L5
Flexor digitorum longus	L5, **S1, S2**
Flexor hallucis longus	L5, **S1, S2**
Abductor hallucis, other small muscles of foot	S1, S2
Sciatic and common peroneal nerves	
Tibialis anterior	**L4**, L5
Extensor digitorum longus	**L5**, S1

(Continued)

Table 12.4 (Continued)

Lower limb	**Spinal roots**
Extensor hallucis longus	**L5**, S1
Extensor digitorum brevis	L5, S1
Peroneus longus	L5, S1
Peroneus brevis	L5, S1

Modified slightly from Medical Research Council. *Aids to the Examination of the Peripheral Nervous System*. 4th Edition 2000. M.D.O'Brien. Elsevier.

Table 12.5 Root supplies of commonly tested sensory nerves

Upper limb	**Root**
Lateral cutaneous nerve of forearm	**C5–6**
Median (stimulate thumb)	**C6**
Superficial radial to snuffbox Median (index finger)	**C6–7**
Median (middle finger)	**C7**
Ulnar (little finger) Dorsal ulnar cutaneous	**C8**
Medial cutaneous nerve of the forearm	**T1**
Lower limb	
Saphenous	**L4**
Superficial peroneal	**L5**
Sural	**S1**

Chapter 13

Anatomy Buster

A reasonable knowledge of peripheral nerve anatomy is required to interpret nerve conduction studies and EMG. It is helpful to recall not only the nerve supply to a muscle, but also the relevant spinal roots and course of the axons through the plexus. The 'Anatomy Buster' is designed with the neurophysiological examination in mind, with diagrams highlighting the myotomes affected with common root and plexus injuries, and the relevant sensory anatomy displayed alongside. See Figs 13.1 to 13.28.

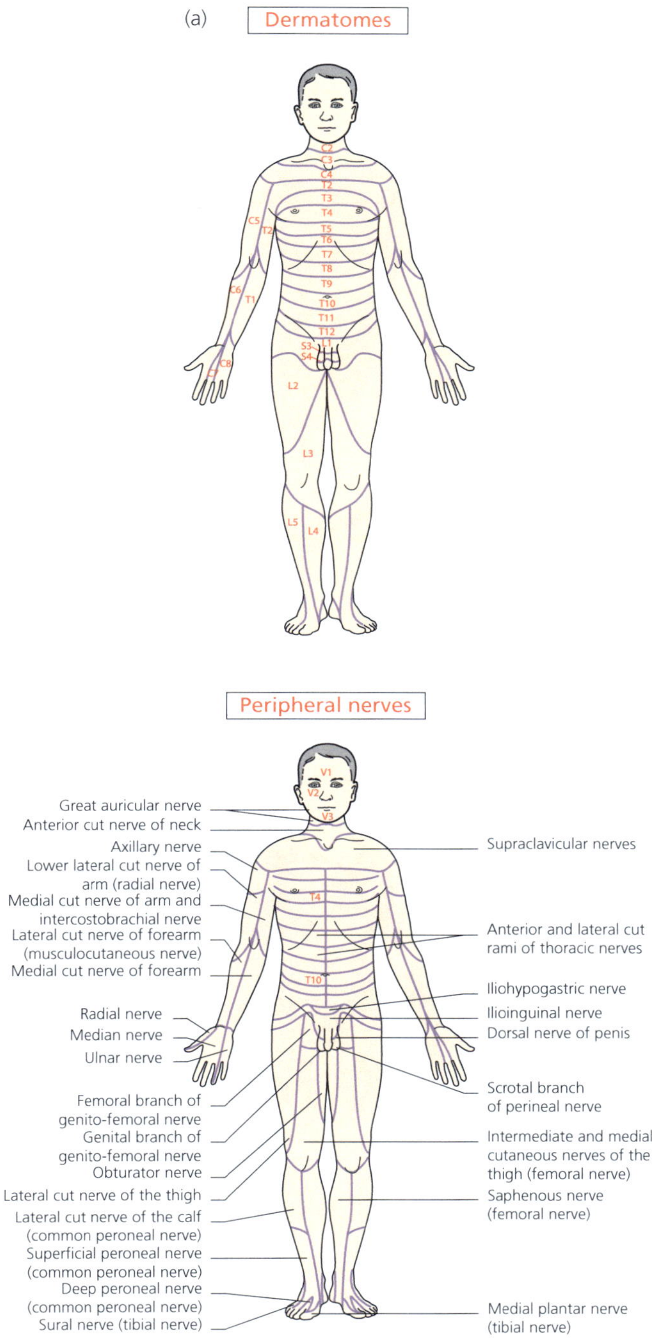

Figure 13.1 Dermatomes and peripheral nerves. (a) Anterior (b) Posterior.

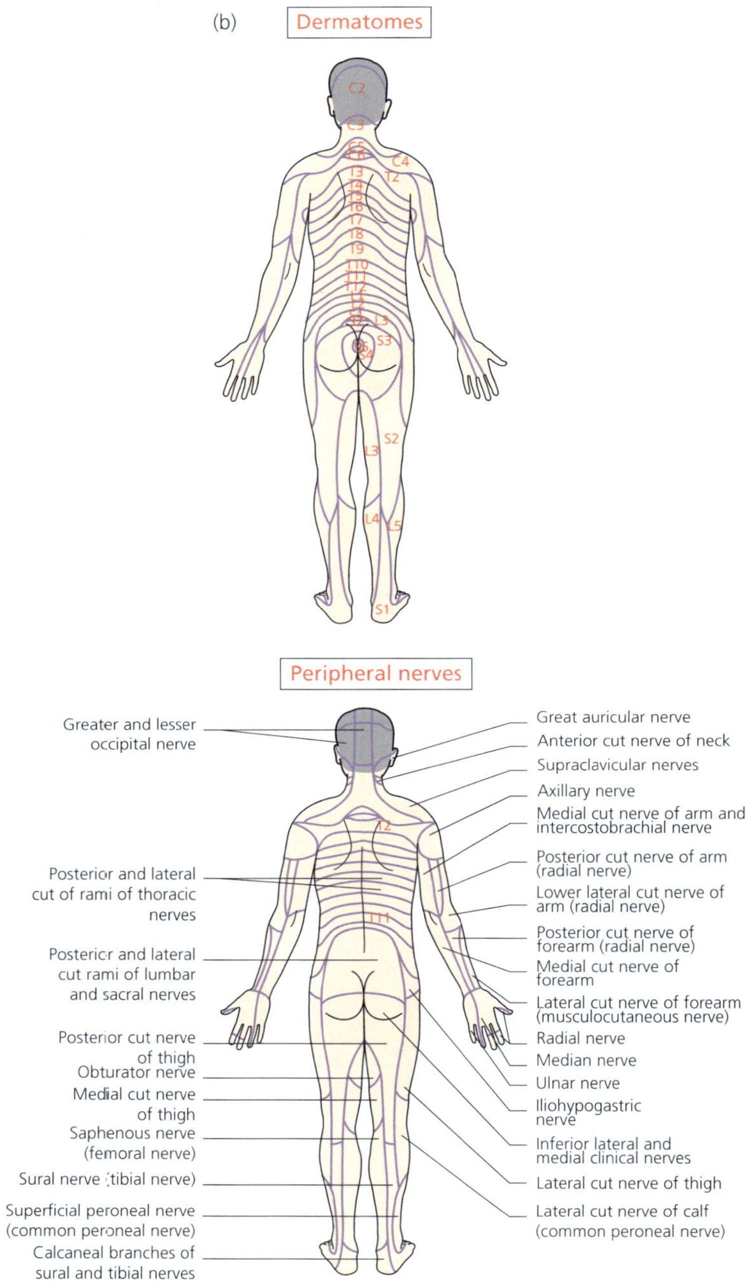

Figure 13.1 (Continued).

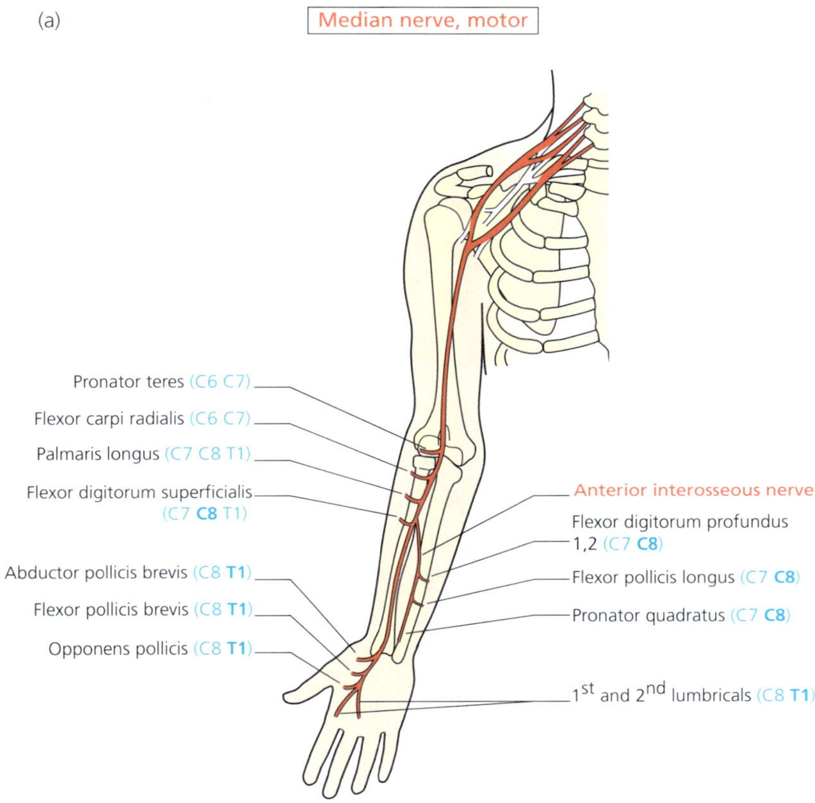

Figure 13.2 Median nerve. (a) Motor (b) Sensory.

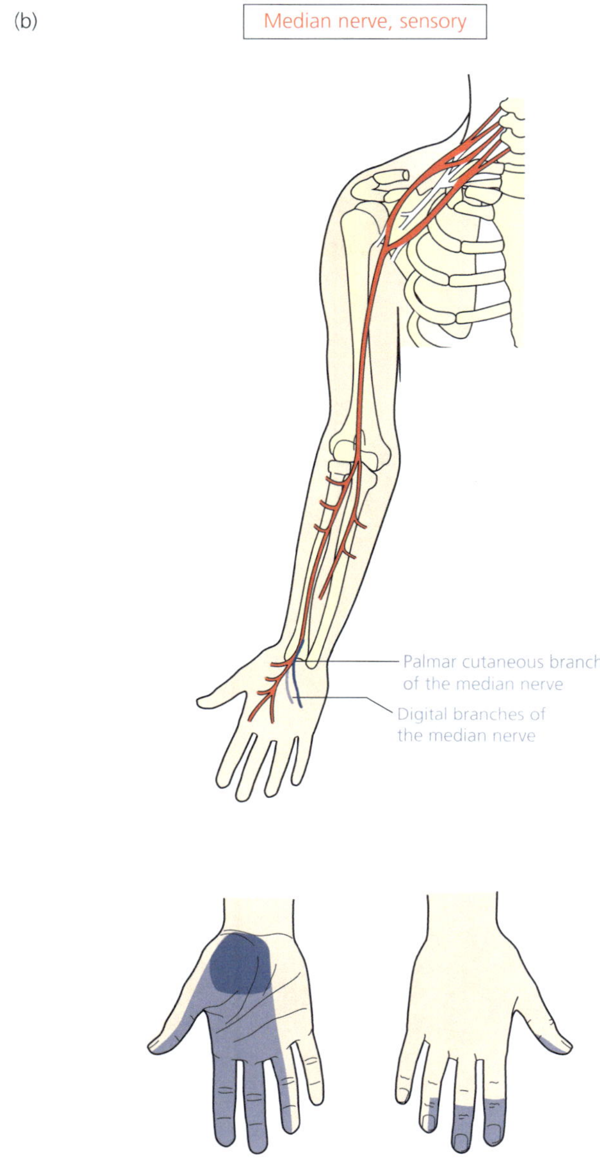

Figure 13.2 (Continued).

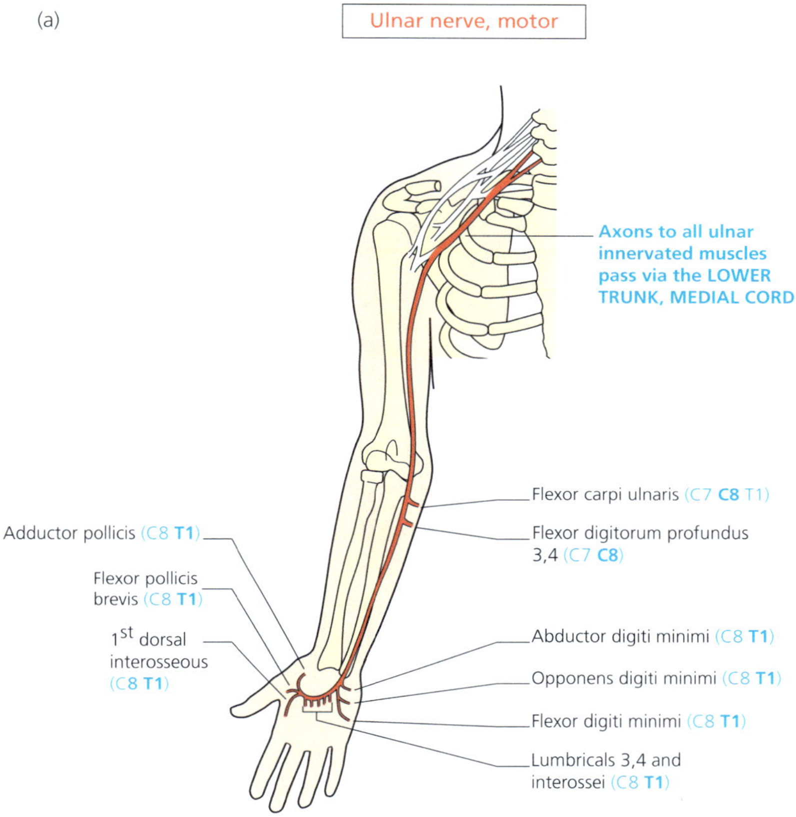

Figure 13.3 Ulnar nerve. (a) Motor (b) Sensory.

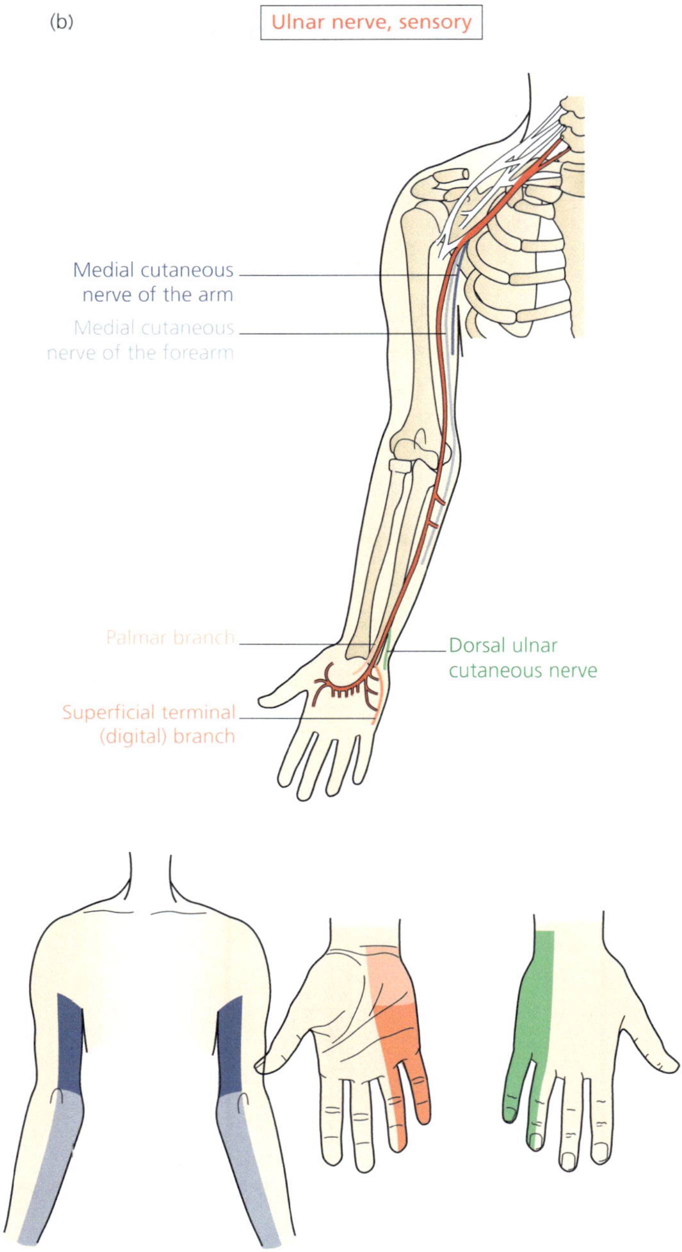

Figure 13.3 (Continued).

(a)

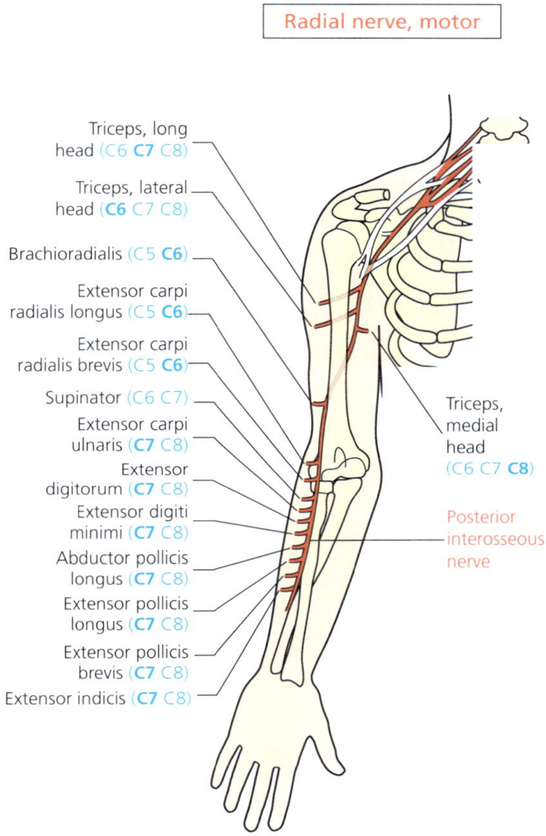

Figure 13.4 Radial nerve. (a) Motor (b) Sensory.

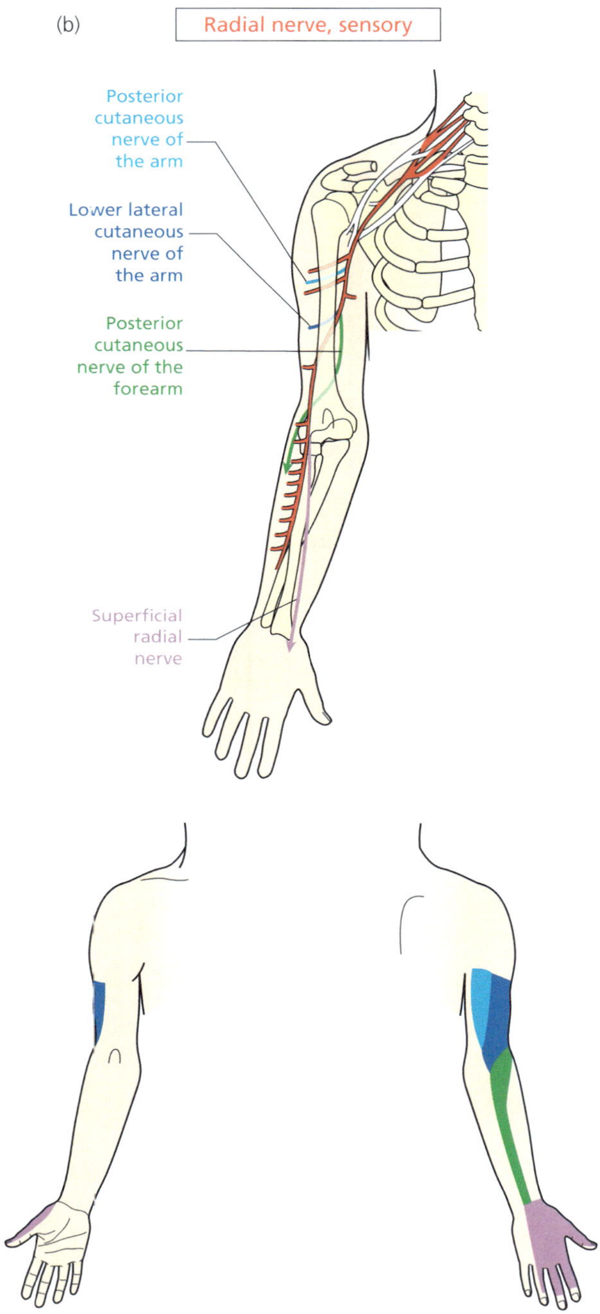

Figure 13.4 (Continued).

(a)

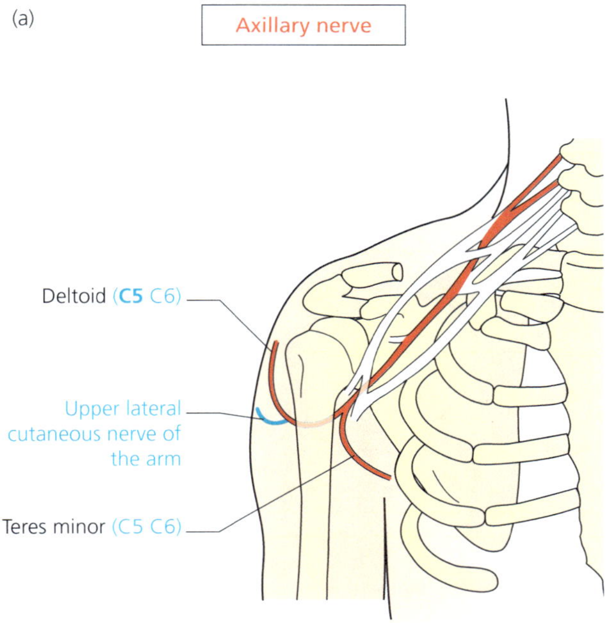

(b)

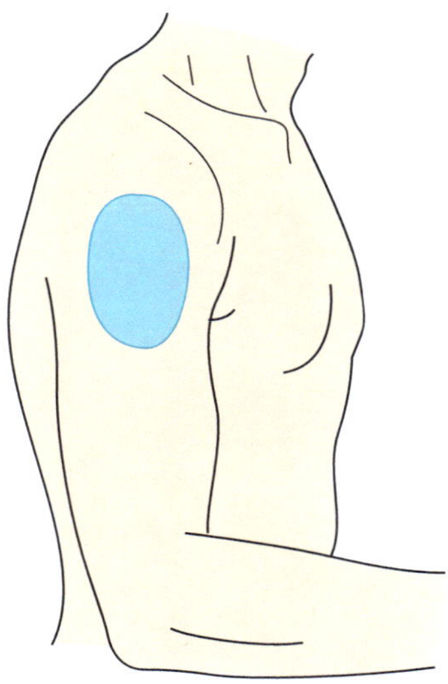

Figure 13.5 Axillary nerve. (a) Motor (b) Sensory.

Long thoracic nerve

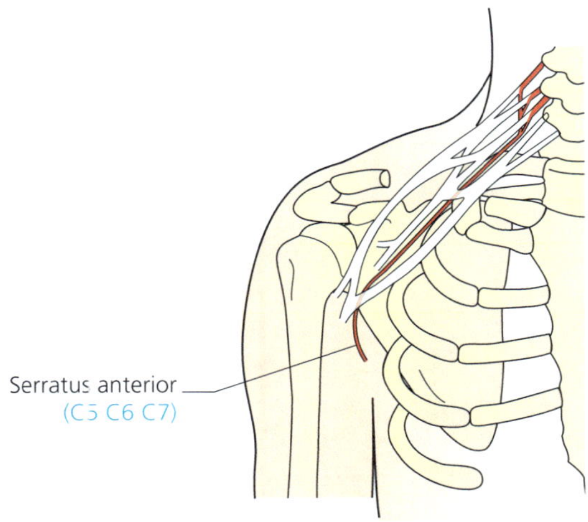

No cutaneous innervation

Figure 13.6 Long thoracic nerve.

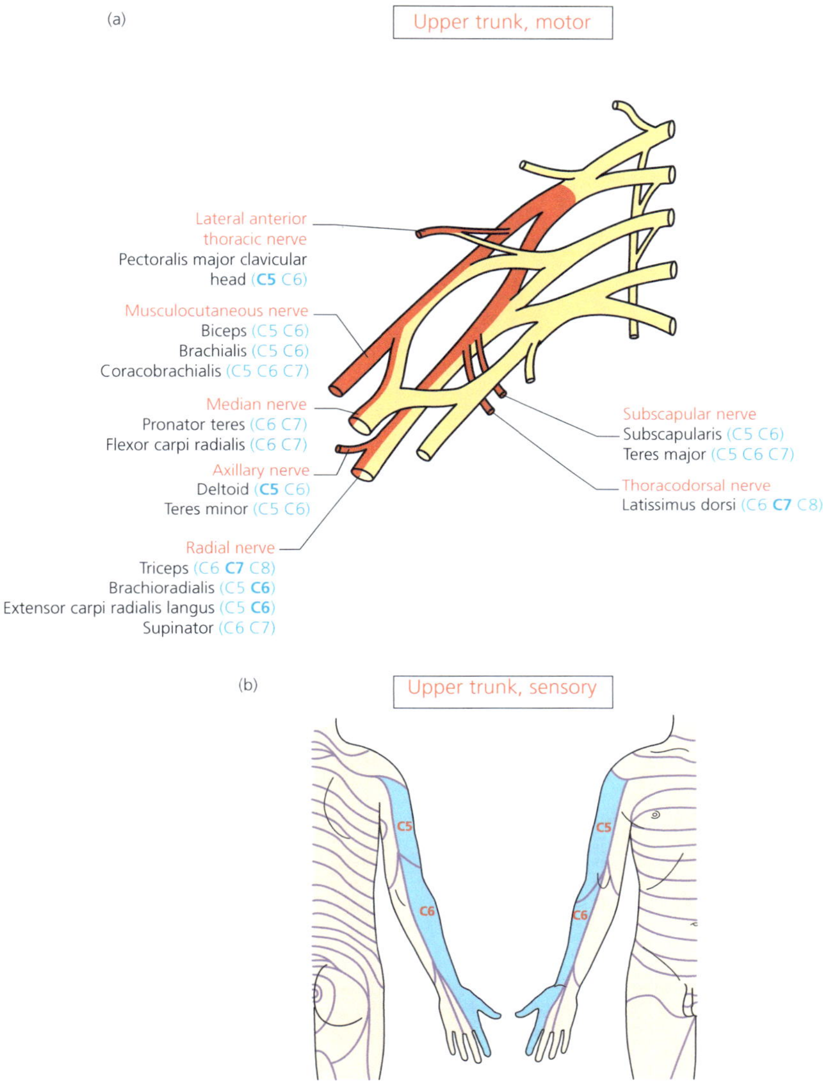

Figure 13.7 Upper trunk brachial plexus lesion. (a) Motor (b) Sensory.

(a)

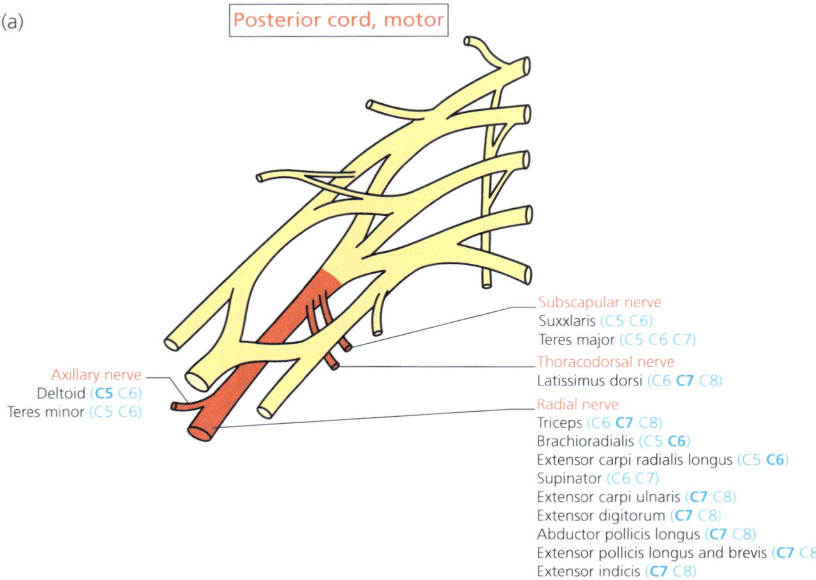

(b)

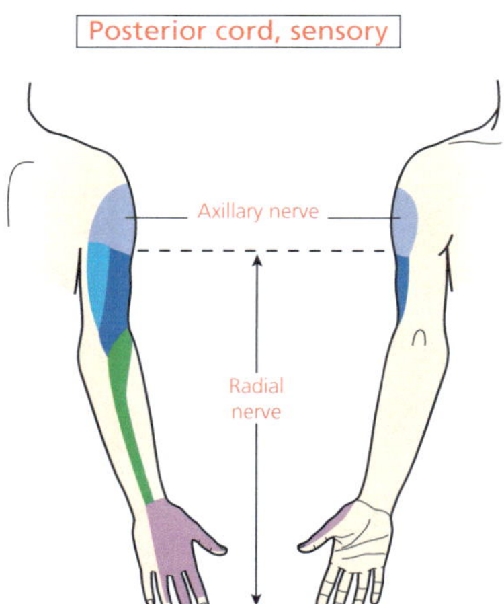

Figure 13.8 Posterior cord brachial plexus lesion. (a) Motor (b) Sensory.

(a)

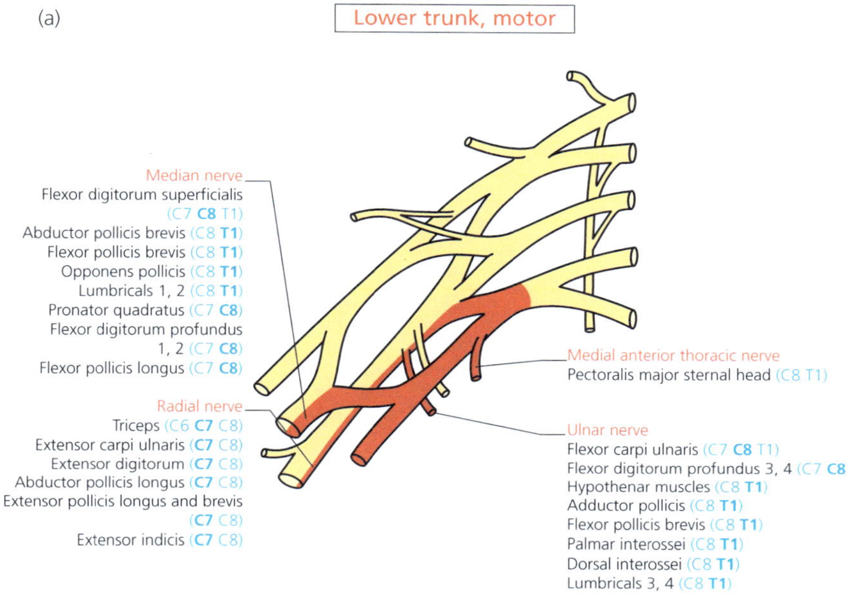

(b)

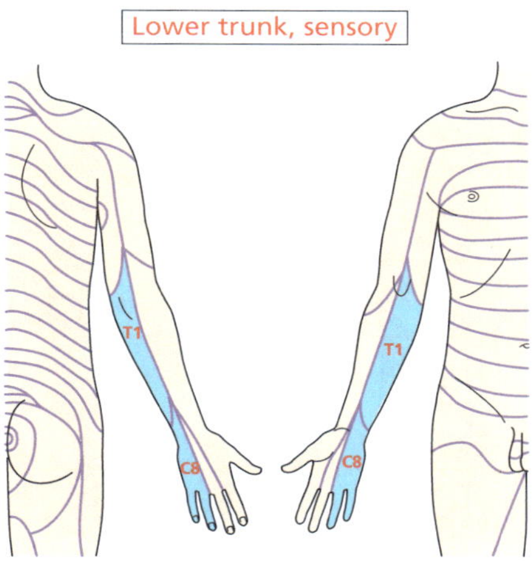

Figure 13.9 Lower trunk brachial plexus lesion. (a) Motor (b) Sensory.

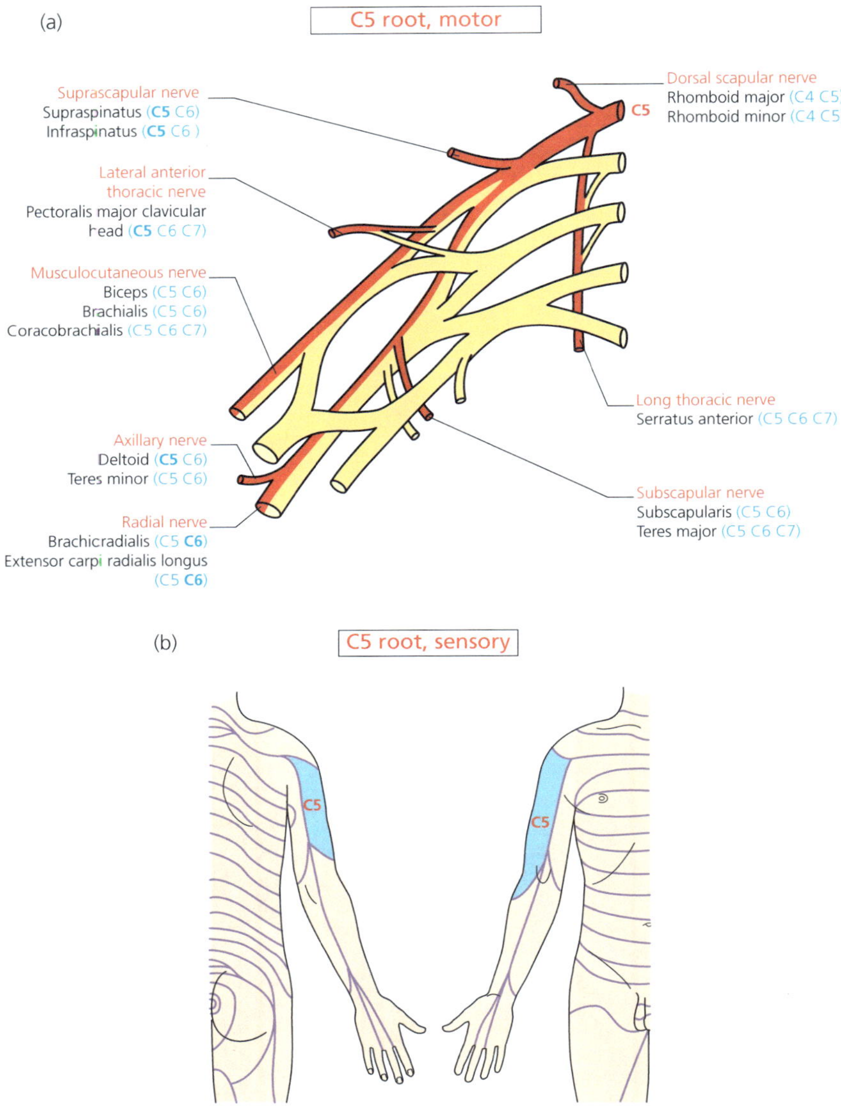

Figure 13.10 C5 root. (a) Motor (b) Sensory.

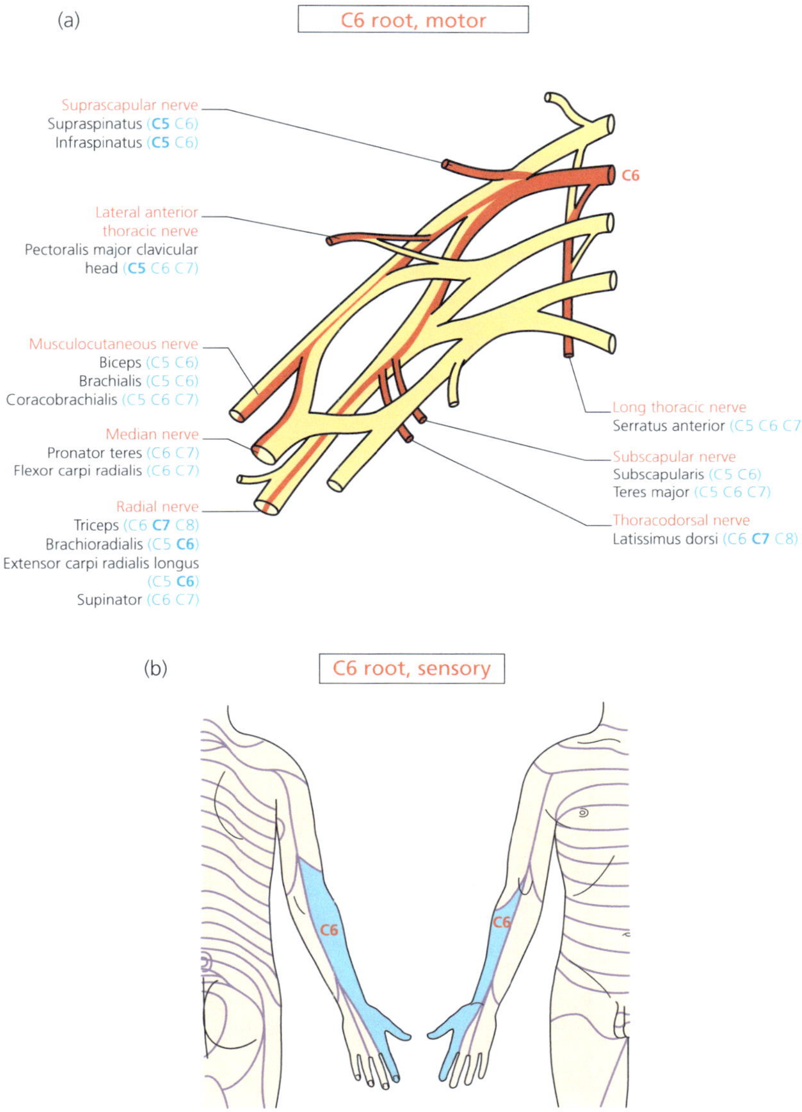

Figure 13.11 C6 root. (a) Motor (b) Sensory.

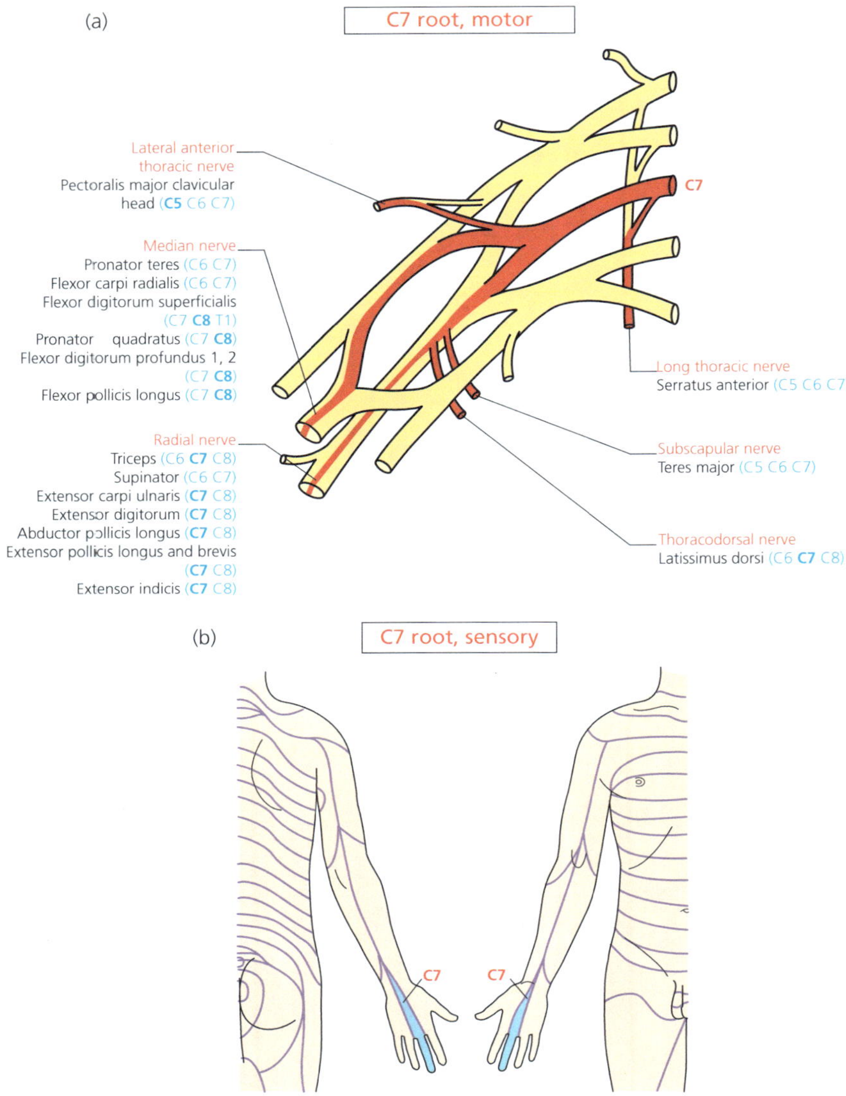

Figure 13.12 C7 root. (a) Motor (b) Sensory.

(a)

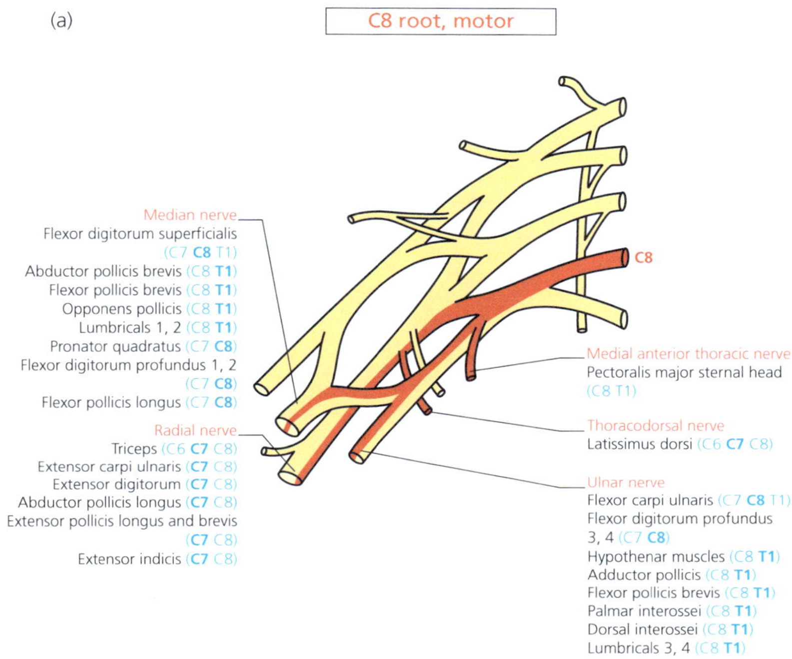

(b)

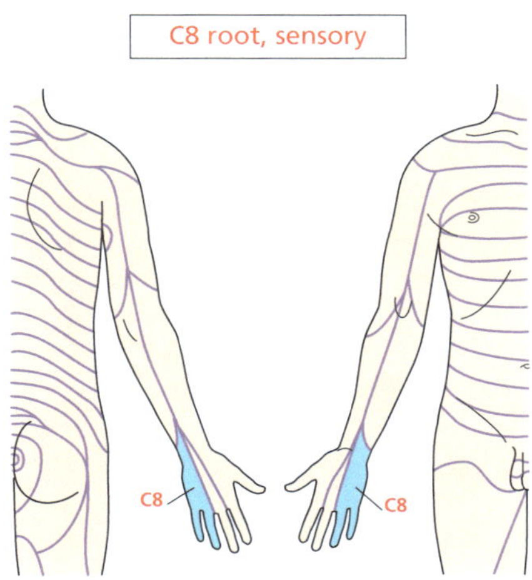

Figure 13.13 C8 root. (a) Motor (b) Sensory.

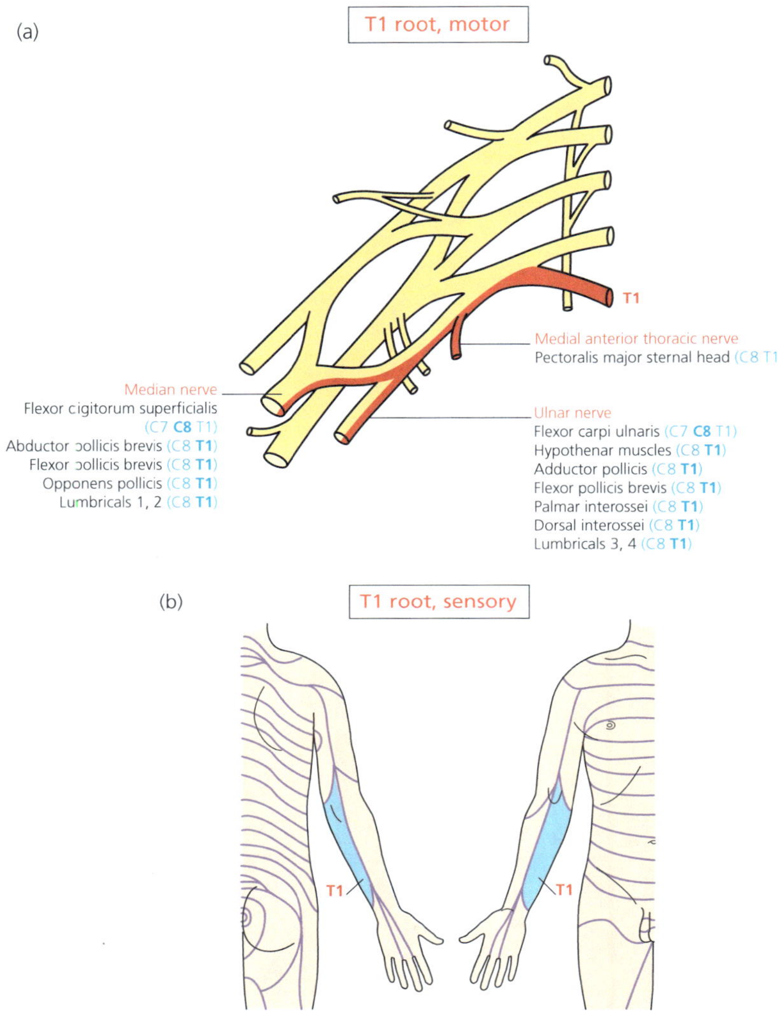

Figure 13.14 T1 root. (a) Motor (b) Sensory.

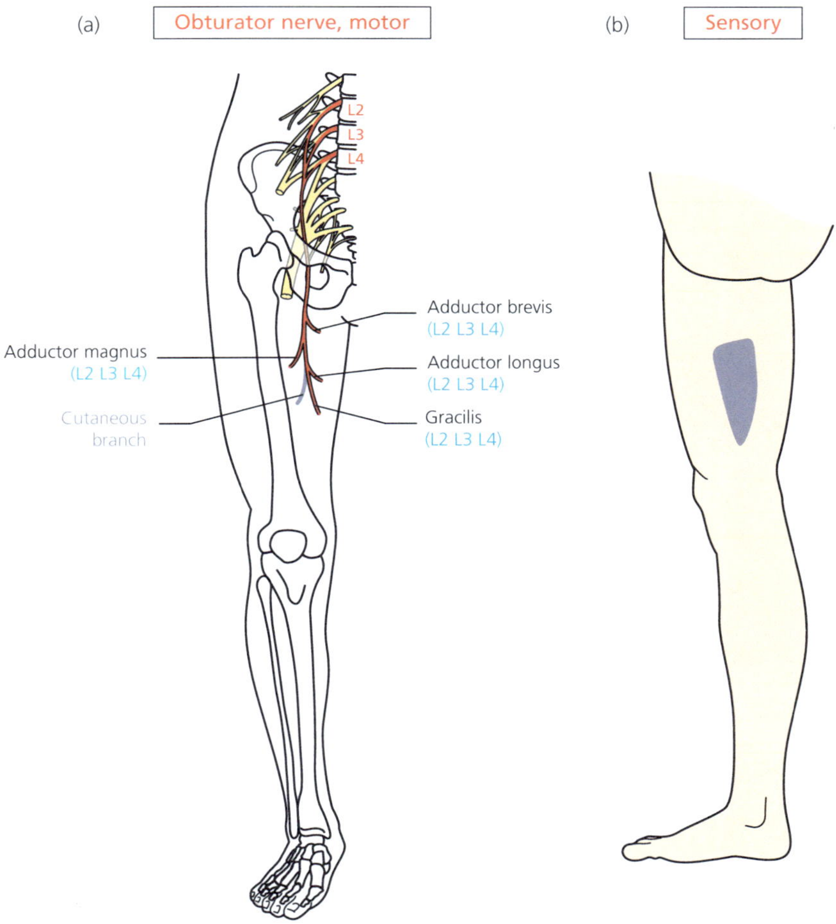

Figure 13.15 Obturator nerve. (a) Motor (b) Sensory.

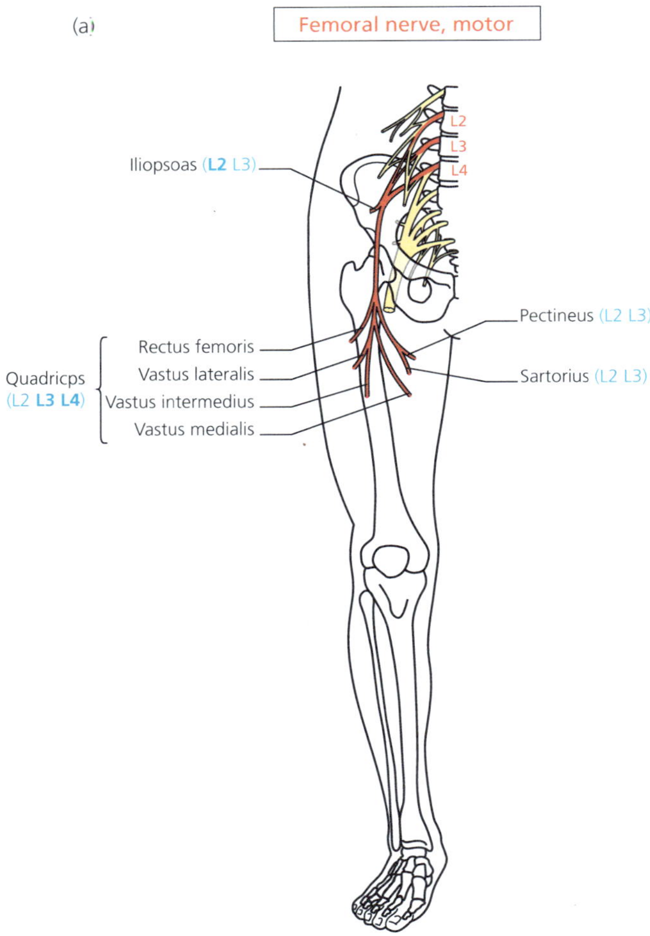

Figure 13.16 (a) Femoral nerve, motor. (b) Femoral nerve, sensory.

(b)

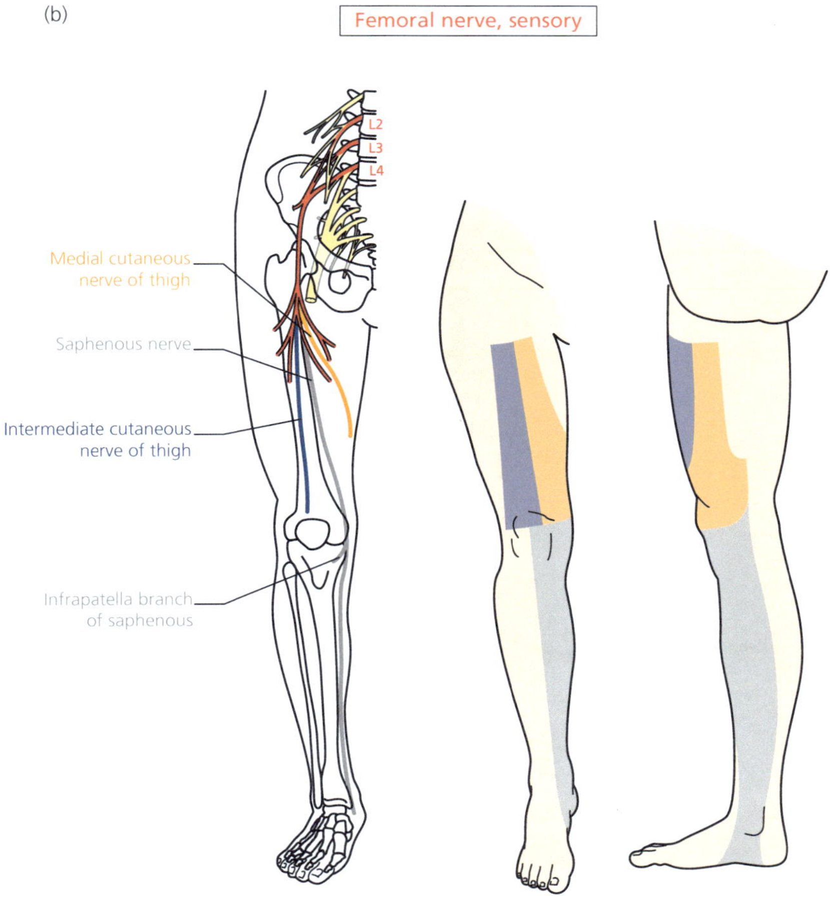

Figure 13.16 (Continued).

(a)

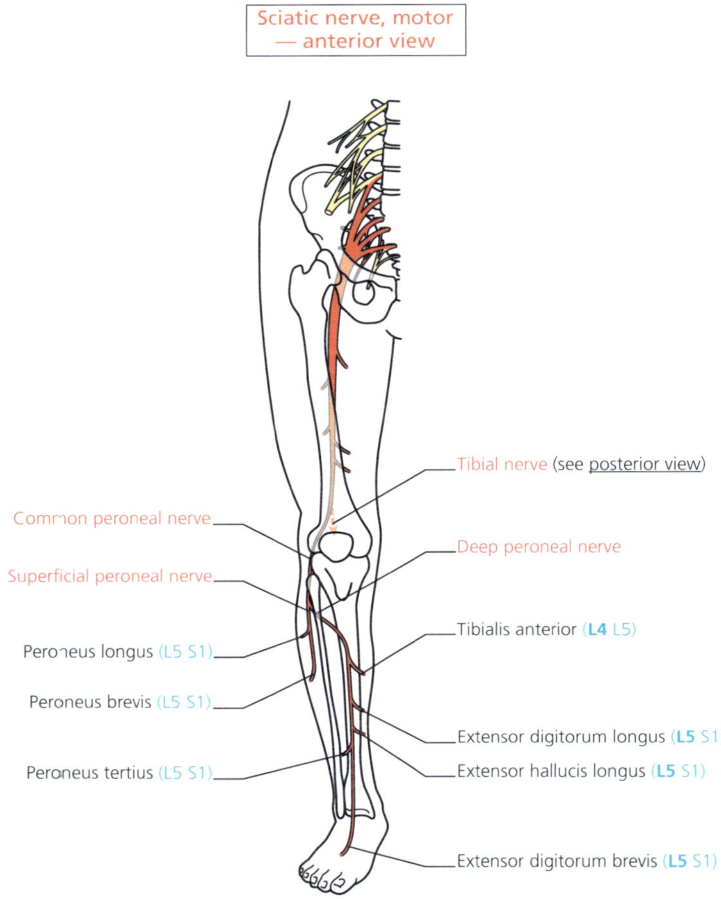

Figure 13.17 (a) Sciatic nerve, motor—anterior view. (b) Sciatic nerve, motor—posterior view.

(b)

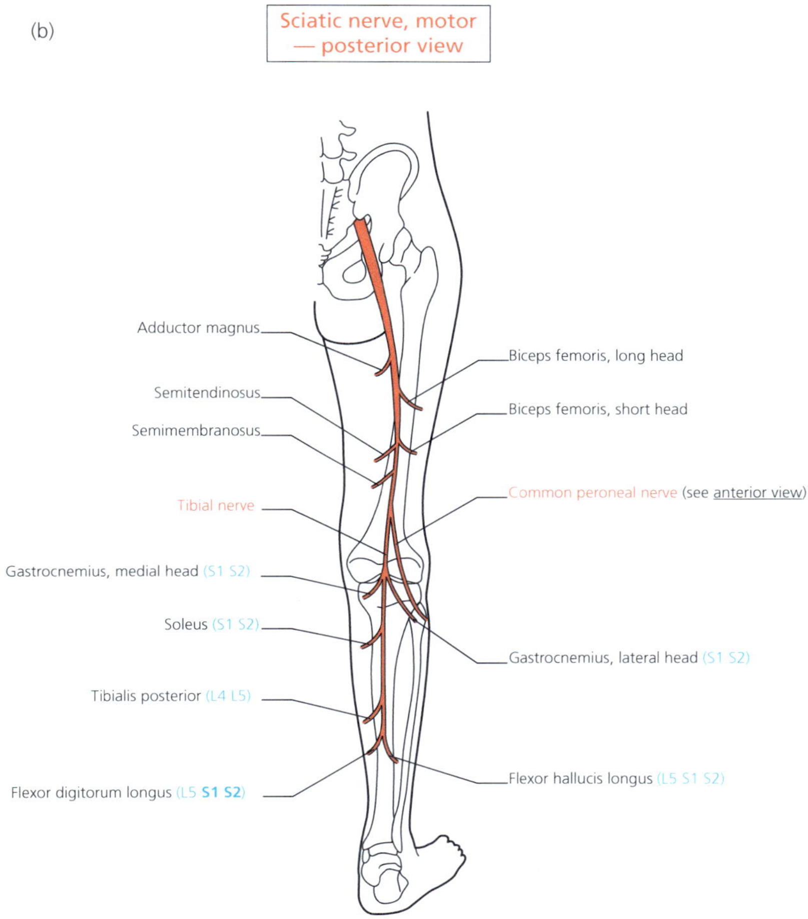

Figure 13.17 (Continued).

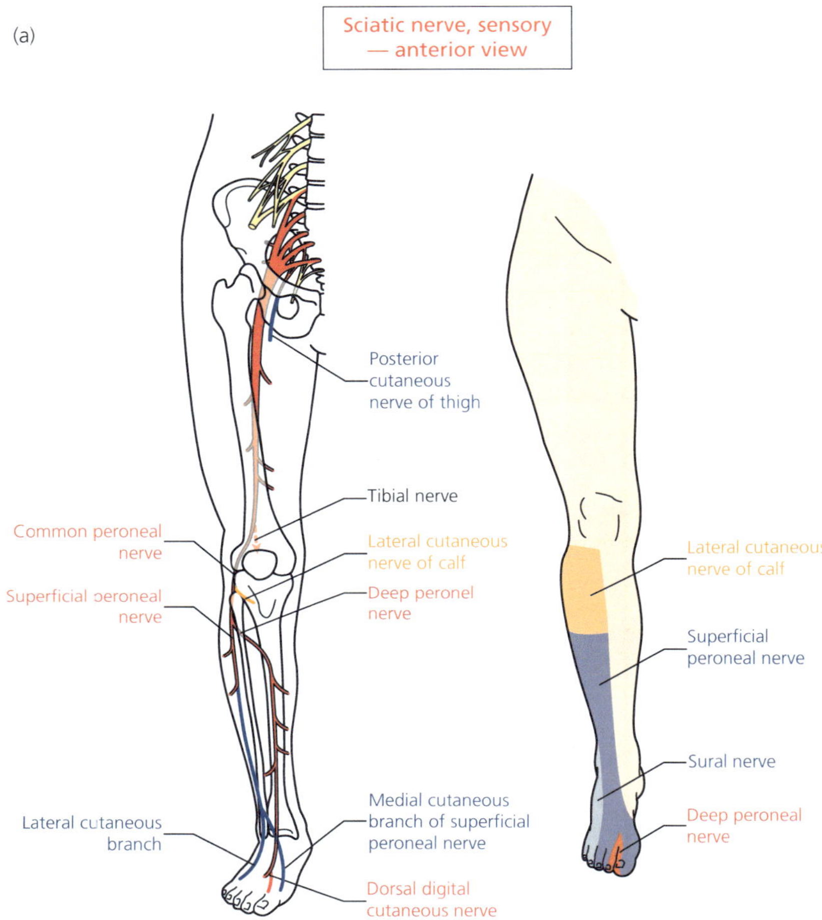

Figure 13.18 (a) Sciatic nerve, sensory—anterior view. (b) Sciatic nerve, sensory—posterior view.

(b)

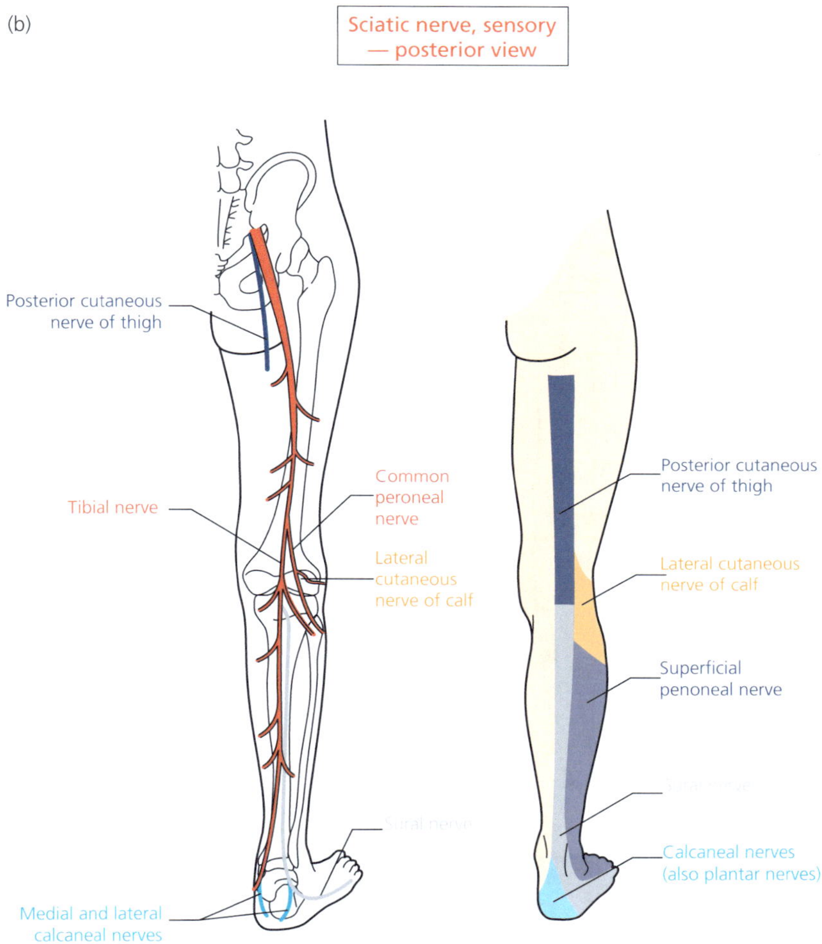

Figure 13.18 (Continued).

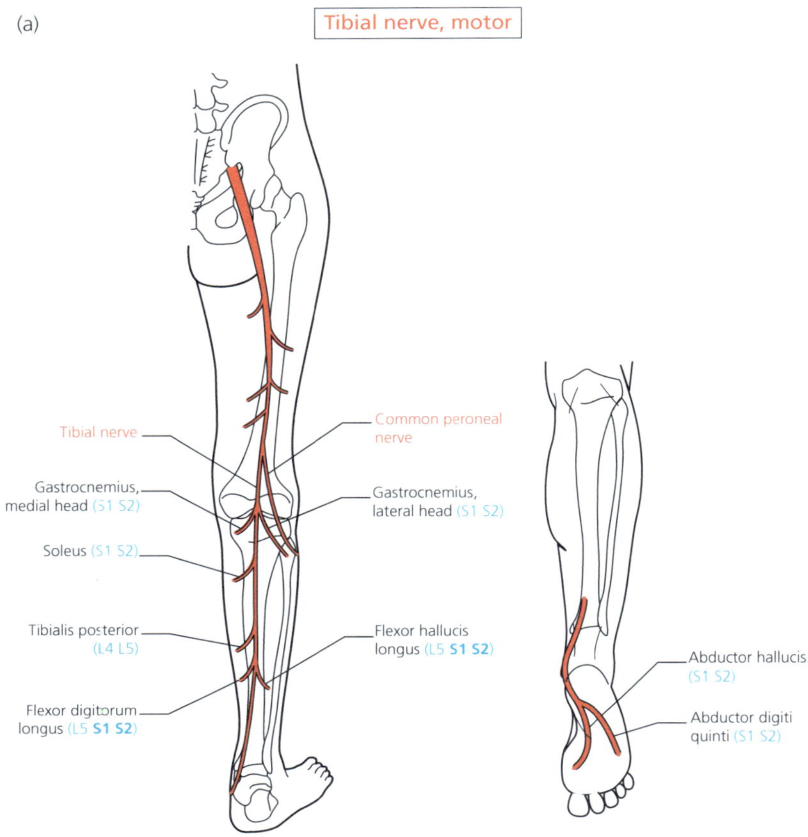

Figure 13.19 (a) Tibial nerve, motor. (b) Tibial nerve, sensory.

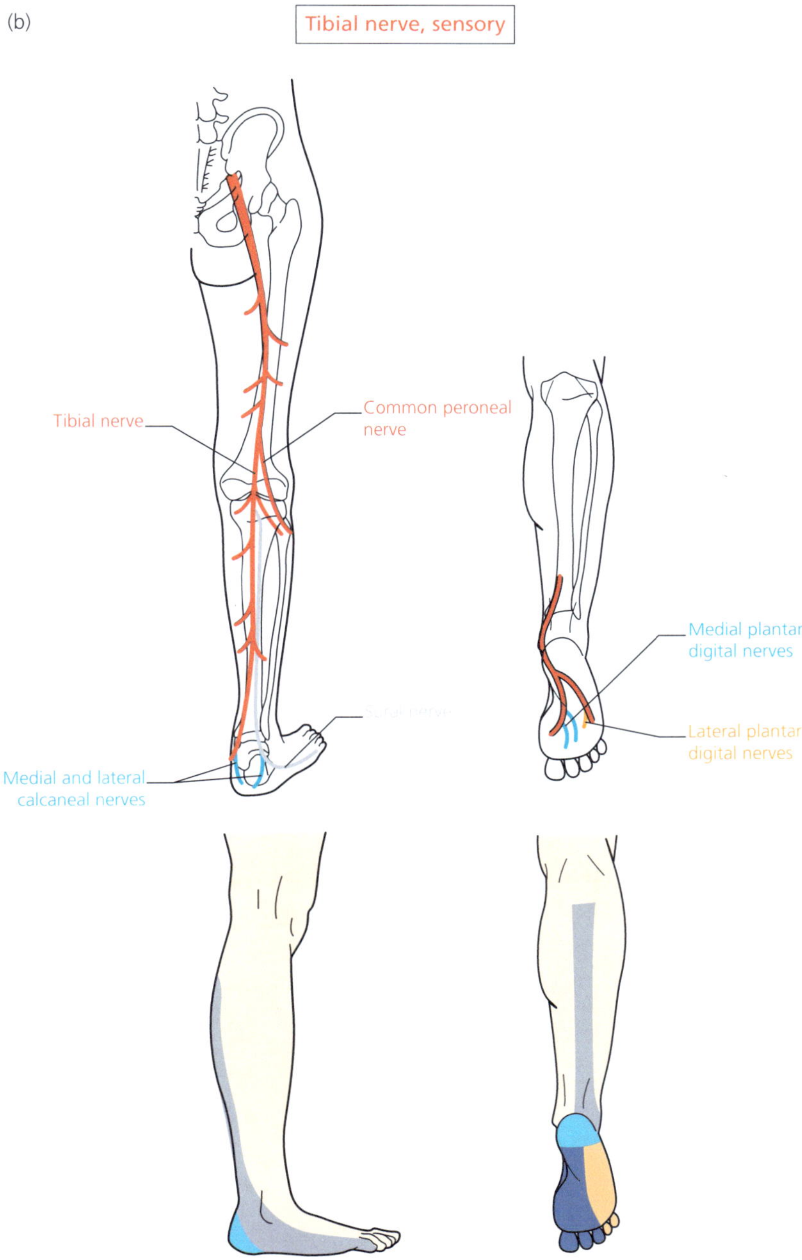

Figure 13.19 (Continued).

(a)

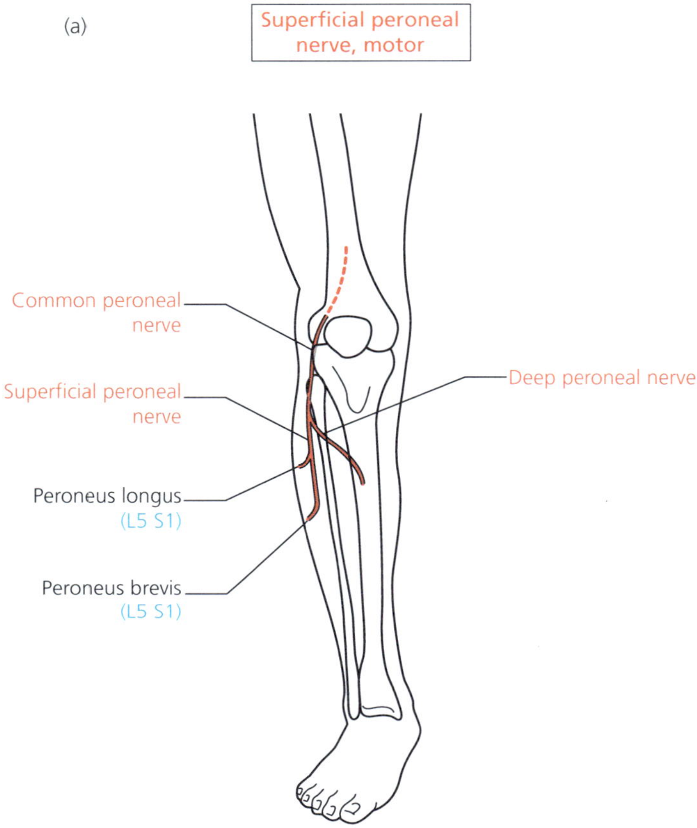

Figure 13.20 (a) Superficial peroneal nerve, motor. (b) Superficial peroneal nerve, sensory.

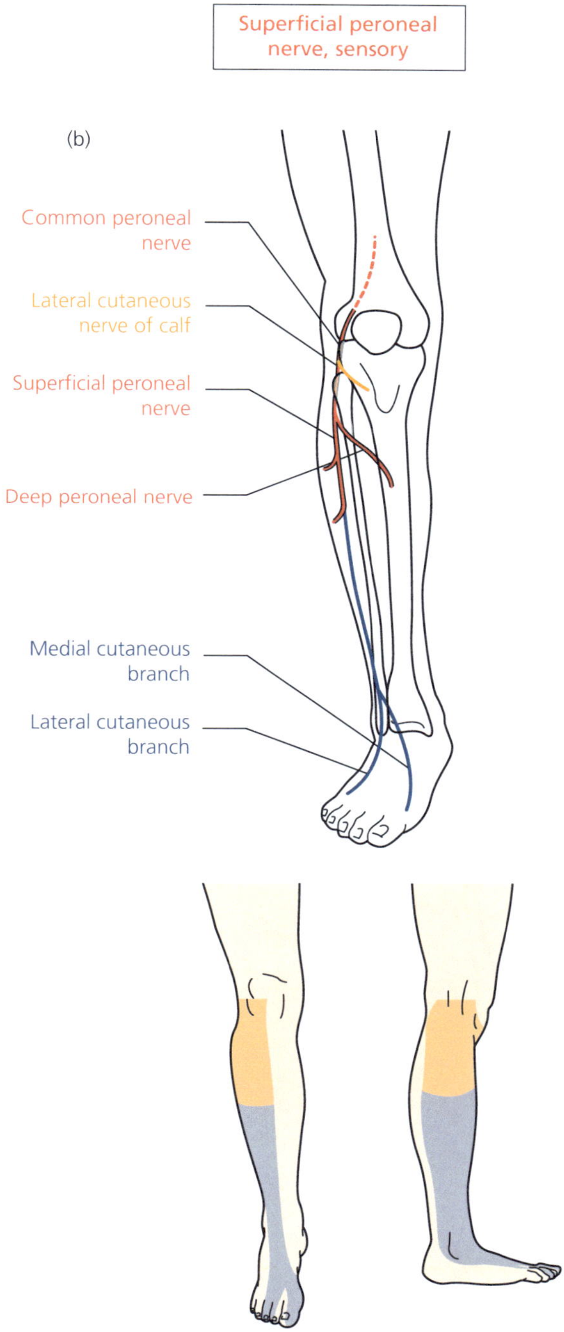

Figure 13.20 (Continued).

(a)

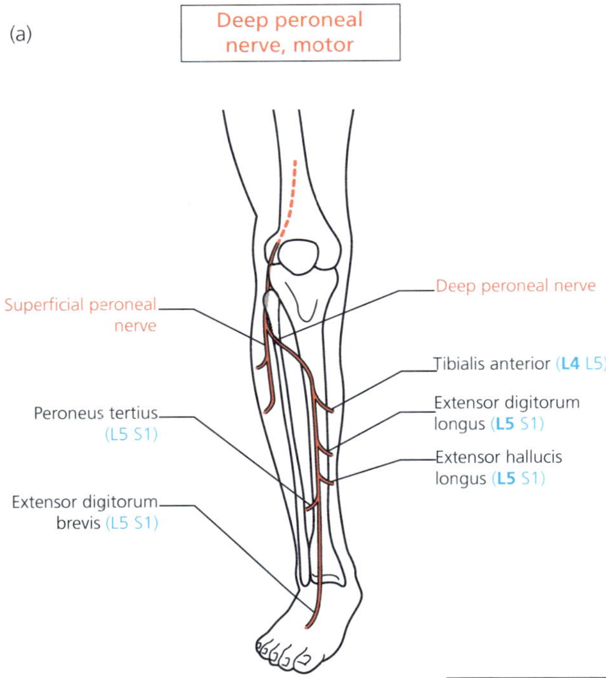

(b)

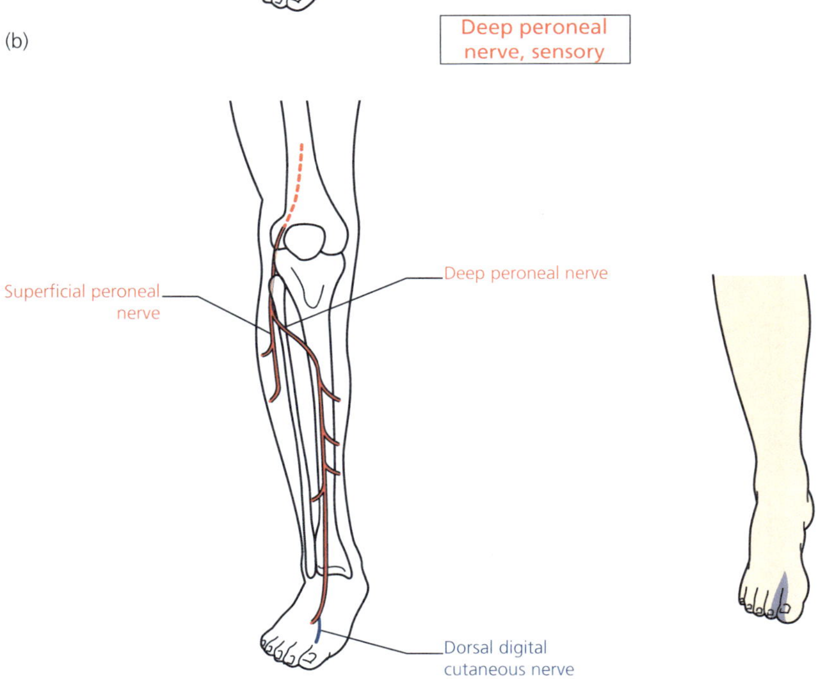

Figure 13.21 (a) Deep peroneal nerve, motor. (b) Deep peroneal nerve, sensory.

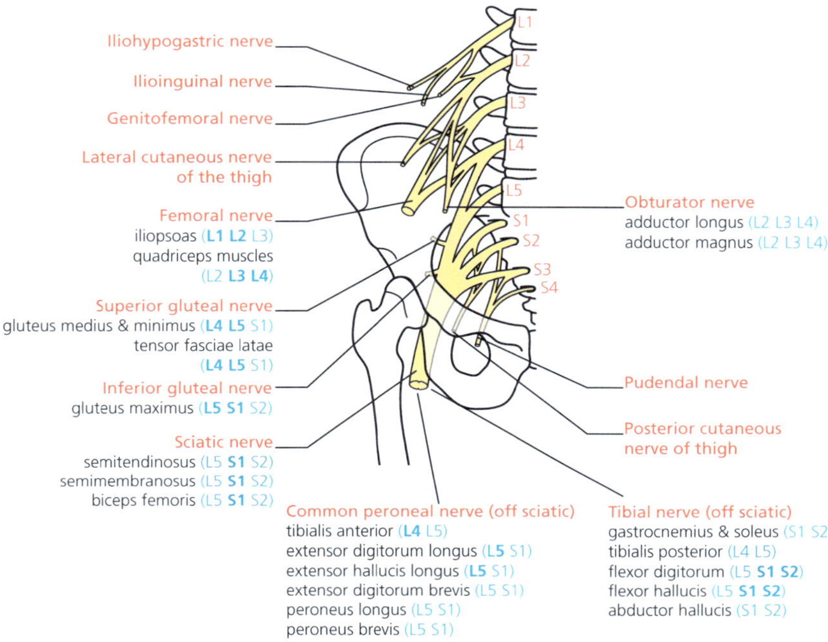

Figure 13.22 Branches of lumbosacral plexus.

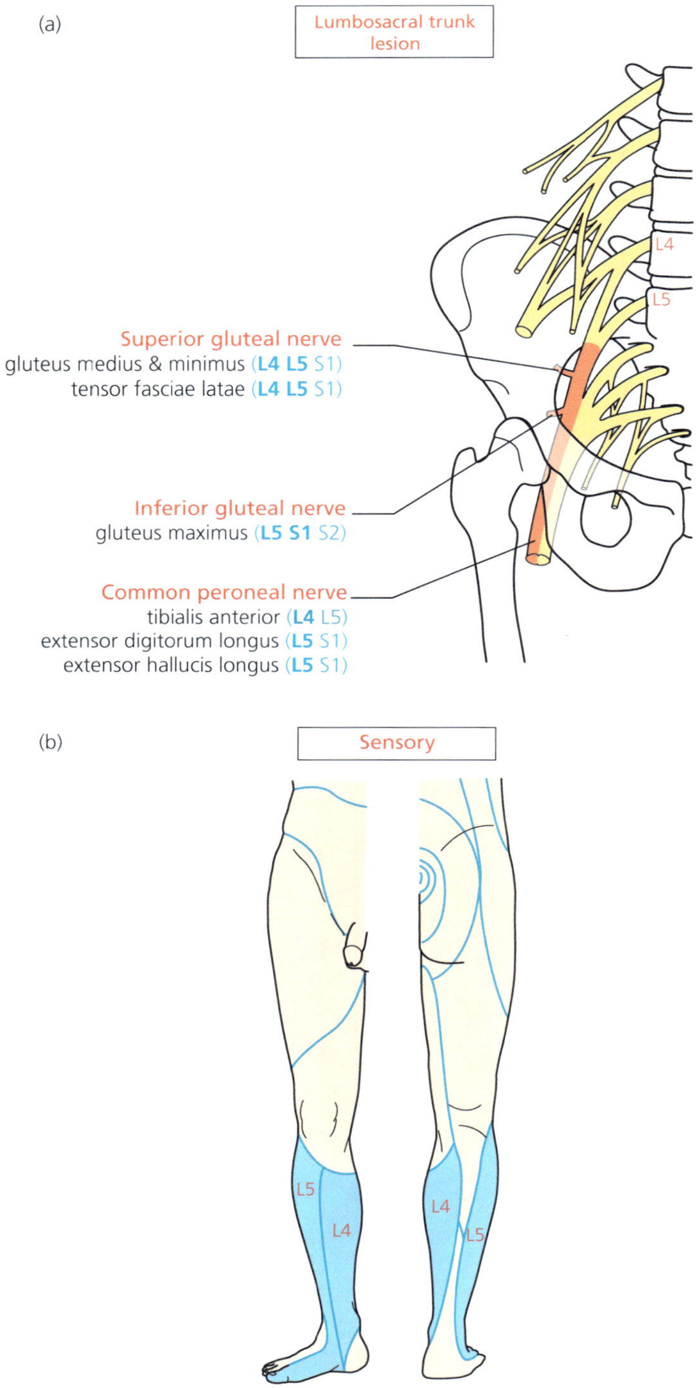

Figure 13.23 Lumbosacral trunk lesion.

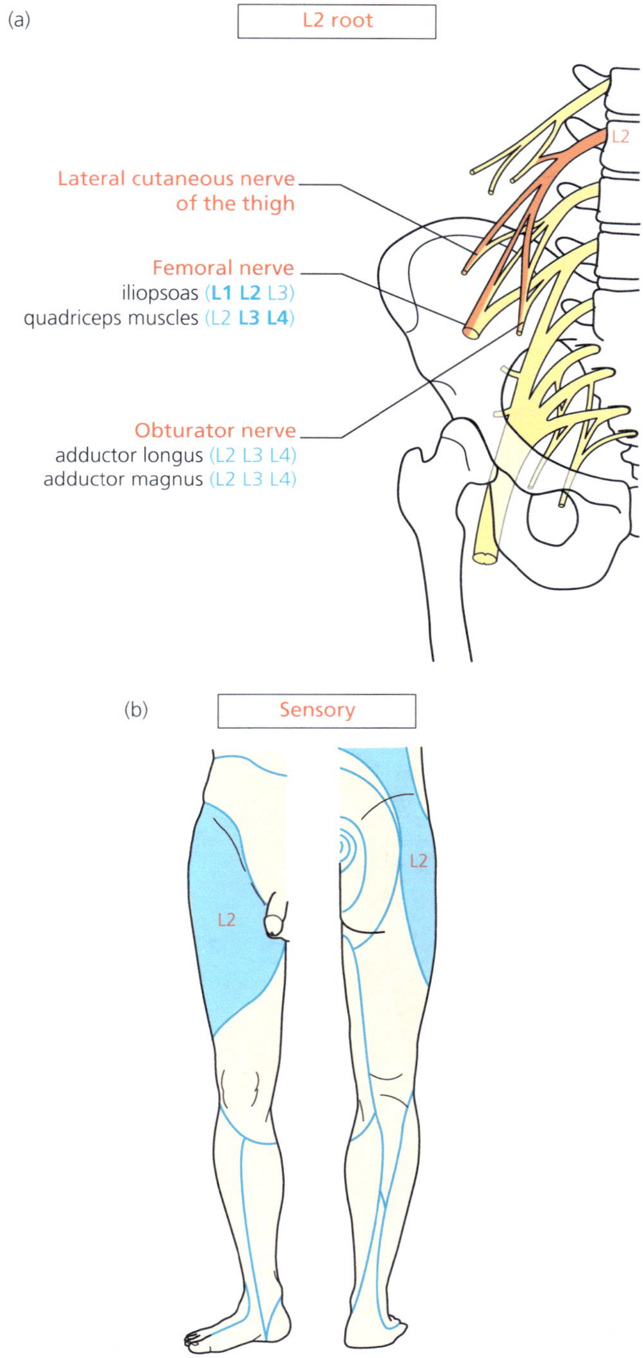

Figure 13.24 L2 root. (a) Motor (b) Sensory.

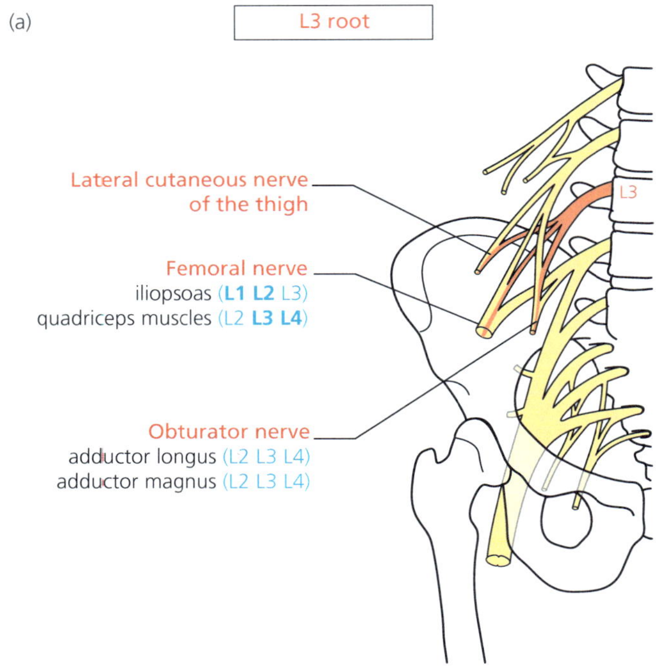

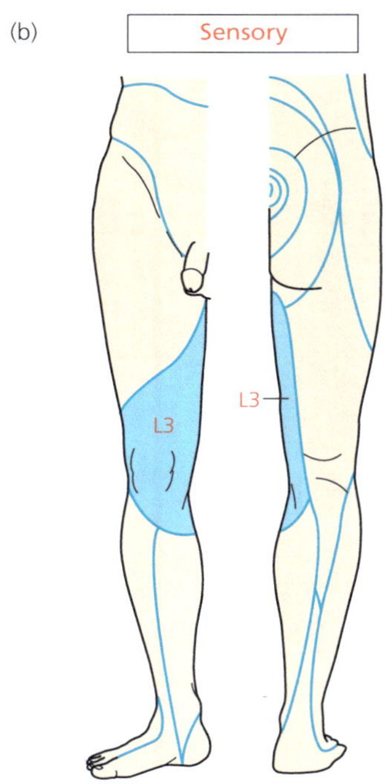

Figure 13.25 L3 root. (a) Motor (b) Sensory.

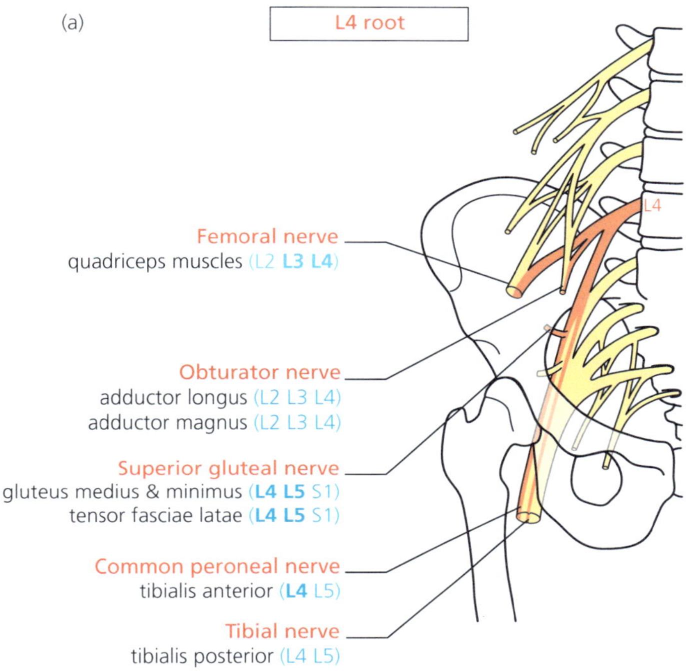

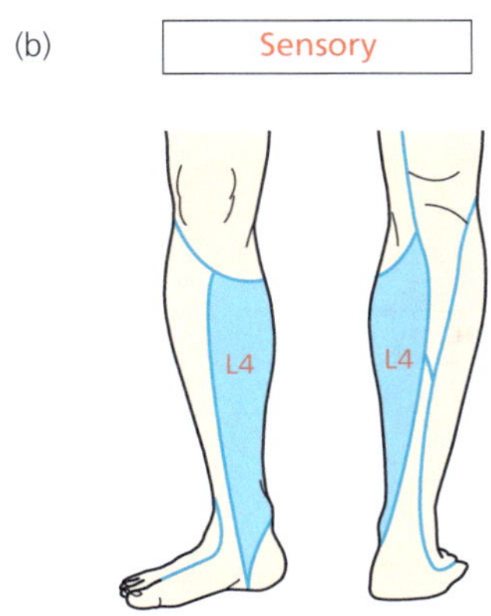

Figure 13.26 L4 root. (a) Motor (b) Sensory.

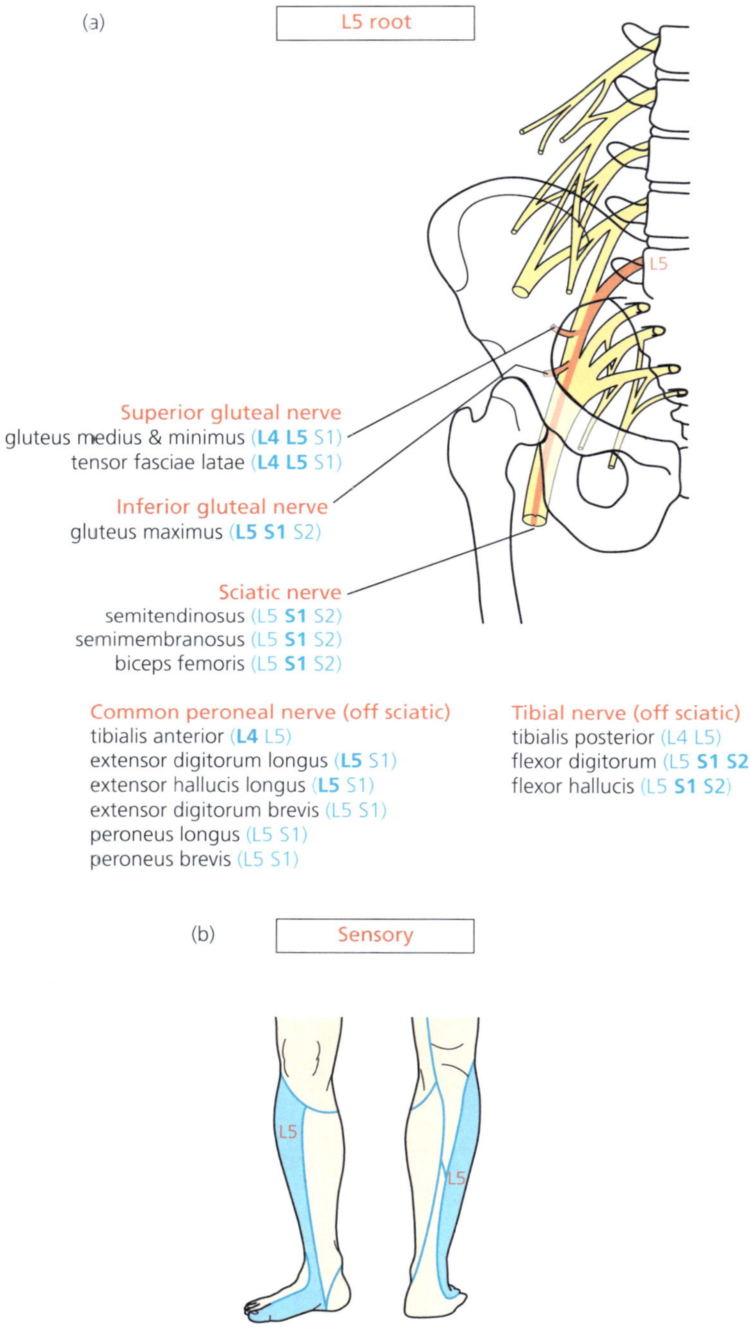

Figure 13.27 L5 root. (a) Motor (b) Sensory.

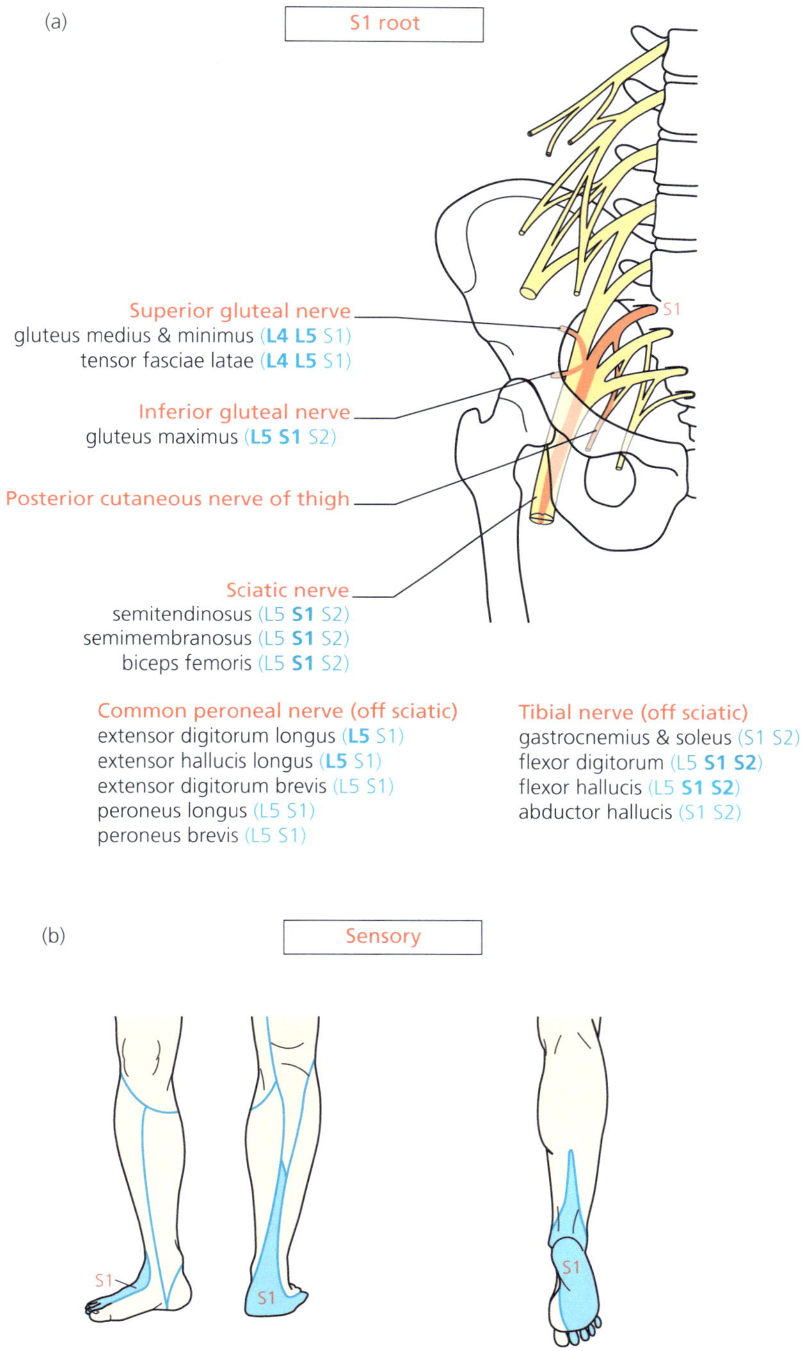

Figure 13.28 S1 root. (a) Motor (b) Sensory.

Section 3

Case Discussions 1–10

Case 1

Clinical presentation

A 47-year-old accountant presents with a 6-month history of painless weakness and wasting of his right hand. He has noted slight weight loss but he has otherwise been well. Examination reveals mild wasting of the right thenar eminence and first dorsal interosseous. Infrequent fasciculations are seen in the right first dorsal interosseous, both deltoids, and right medial gastrocnemius. Deep tendon reflexes from the right upper and lower limb are brisk compared to the left, but both plantar responses remain flexor. Sensation is objectively normal. The patient has consulted the referring neurologist twice, who now suspects motor neuron disease in light of the clinical progression. For results of nerve conduction studies and EMG see Tables 14.1 and 14.2.

Questions

1. Does the neurophysiology support a diagnosis of amyotrophic lateral sclerosis?
2. What do you make of the conduction findings in the right median nerve?

Interpretation

Sensory response amplitudes are almost all normal, suggesting that there is minimal if any sensory axon loss distal to the dorsal root ganglion. Right upper limb motor responses are mildly low amplitude, which suggests the slight wasting and weakness of these muscles is likely to be due to partial axon loss.

An important differential diagnosis for asymmetrical upper limb weakness without sensory loss is multifocal motor neuropathy with conduction block,

Table 14.1 Nerve conduction studies

Nerve	Stimulation	Recording	Amplitude (μV or mV)			Onset latency (ms)			Conduction velocity (m/s)			F wave latency (ms)		
			R	L	N	R	L	N	R	L	N	R	L	N
Sensory														
Median	Index finger	Wrist	6	12	**≥7**				37	58	**≥49**			
Ulnar	Little finger	Wrist	6	6	**≥5**				50	53	**≥49**			
Radial	Forearm	Snuff box	28		**≥12**				63		**≥50**			
Sural	Calf	Posterior ankle	17	15	**≥10**				43	35	**≥40**			
Superficial peroneal	Lateral ankle	Dorsum of foot	10		**≥5**				39		**≥40**			
Motor														
Median	Wrist	APB	3.7	6.5	**≥4**	4.8	3.8	**≤4.2**				30	28	**≤31**
	Elbow	APB	3.7	6.3					48	54	**≥49**			
Ulnar	Wrist	ADM	5.4	9.8	**≥6**	2.7	2.7	**≤3.3**				29	29	**≤32**
	Below elbow	ADM	5.5	9.8					54	55	**≥49**			
	Above elbow	ADM	5.0	9.6					53	55	**≥49**			
	Axilla	ADM	4.9	9.6					58	59	**≥49**			
	Erb's	ADM	4.5	9.0										
	Cervical	ADM	4.1											

Tibial	Ankle	AH	6.7	≥**4**	4.6	≤**5.8**			54	≤**56**
	Knee	AH	6.0				43	≥**41**		
Peroneal	Ankle	EDB	3.7	≥**2**	3.9	≤**6.5**				≤**56**
	Fibular head	EDB	3.7				42	≥**41**		
	Popliteal fossa	EDB	3.8				44			

Sensory amplitudes are μV, motor amplitudes mV. R, right; L, left; N, normal; APB, abductor pollicis brevis; ADM, abductor digiti minimi; AH, abductor hallucis brevis; EDB extensor digitorum brevis.

Table 14.2 EMG

Muscle	Spontaneous activity	Motor unit action potential			Recruitment	Interference pattern
		Duration	Amplitude	Phases		
R 1st dorsal interosseous	2+ fibs	↑	↑↑	↑↑	Reduced	↓↓
R abductor pollicis brevis	Nil	↑	↑↑	↑↑	Reduced	↓↓
R deltoid	Nil	↑	↑	↑	Reduced	↓↓
R biceps	Fascics	↑	↑	N	Reduced	↓
L deltoid	Fascics	↑	N	↑	Reduced	↓
R vastus medialis	1+ fibs	↑	↑	↑↑	Reduced	↓
R rectus femoris	Nil	N	↑	N	N	N
R adductor longus	1+ fibs	↑	↑	↑	Reduced	↓
R tibialis anterior	Fascics, 1+ fibs	↑	↑↑	↑	Reduced	↓
R medial gastrocnemius	Fascics	↑	N	N	Poor activation	↓
L vastus medialis	2+ fibs	↑	N	↑	Reduced	↓
R rectus abdominus	Nil	↑	↑	↑	Reduced	↓
Tongue	No full relaxation	N	N	N	N	N

↑, mildly increased; ↑↑, moderately increased; ↓, mildly decreased; ↓↓, moderately decreased; R, right; L, left; N, normal; fascics, fasciculation potentials; fibs, fibrillation potentials.

a well-known mimic of amyotrophic lateral sclerosis in this setting. However, in this example even ulnar nerve stimulation at cervical root level revealed no motor conduction block to the weak right abductor digiti minimi muscle. This fits with clinical expectation since the mild wasting and small CMAP from that muscle suggest weakness is due to partial motor axon loss not conduction block (which causes weakness without wasting).

EMG findings are consistent with moderate severity partial denervation of the weak hand muscles with small CMAPs, confirming axon loss. There are also findings suggesting milder partial denervation of some clinically unaffected muscles. This denervation affects muscles innervated by different nerves originating from the same spinal level, and affects multiple different levels within the cervical, thoracic, and lumbosacral regions of the spinal cord.

Thus the neurophysiological examination shows that the pathological process results in loss of motor axons, and the relative normality of sensory responses suggests it is likely to be preganglionic (proximal to the dorsal root ganglion), either at the level of the anterior horn cells or, far less likely, affecting multiple motor roots. This latter possibility is highly unlikely given the presentation and age of the patient, and MRI of the spine subsequently showed no evidence of motor root pathology, so is in keeping with the neurophysiological suspicion of anterior horn cell disease.

Although there is no EMG evidence of denervation in the bulbar region, in this clinical context the neurophysiological examination is in keeping with the clinical suspicion of motor neuron disease. Other motor neuronopathies deserve mention since they could potentially cause similar neurophysiological findings, albeit with a different presentation. There is a reasonable amount of spontaneous EMG activity at rest, which is common in conditions with active ongoing motor unit remodelling, such as motor neuron disease. Generally there are fewer fibrillation potentials or positive sharp waves in chronic motor neuronopathies, although they may still occur. In chronic conditions, motor unit action potentials are likely to be long duration and high amplitude, whereas in relatively early active disease they are more likely to be polyphasic and accompanied by fibrillation potentials because of the ongoing remodelling of motor units.

The slowing of median sensory conduction across the right wrist plus slight reduction of sensory response amplitude (compared to the left) are common incidental findings. Together with prolongation of the distal **motor latency** to the right abductor pollicis brevis, they suggest a median neuropathy at the wrist. In this case it is asymptomatic, so the patient does not have carpal tunnel syndrome. Its importance is its recognition, such that it may be discounted from further discussion.

Conclusion

The neurophysiological examination provides support for the clinical suspicion of motor neuron disease, with evidence of denervation in three out of four spinal segments, but not the bulbar muscles. There is an incidental finding of an asymptomatic moderate severity right median neuropathy at the wrist.

Comment: neurophysiology and the diagnosis of motor neuron disease

1. *The diagnosis of motor neuron disease is clinical.* Although supporting evidence is provided by the neurophysiological examination, the referring neurologist makes the diagnosis based on an appropriate history and combination of upper and lower motor neuron examination findings. The neurophysiology is particularly helpful in ruling out mimicking conditions such as multifocal motor neuropathy with conduction block, and in detecting more extensive denervation than is clinically apparent, thus helping to make an early diagnosis. Because of the implications of the diagnosis, the EMG should not be overinterpreted, and a repeat study should be performed if necessary to look for disease progression.

2. *Do not over interpret fasciculations.* Fasciculations found in isolation, without other EMG evidence of denervation, are not necessarily pathological. For example, they may be widespread in benign cramp-fasciculation syndrome, but there is no supporting EMG evidence of denervation such as fibrillation potentials, alteration in motor unit action potential morphology, or abnormality of recruitment. Furthermore, since there is no denervation these patients do not have muscle wasting or progressive weakness. It is essential that a diagnosis of motor neuron disease is only made in the appropriate clinical context, and that neurophysiological findings are not misinterpreted.

3. *The four spinal regions.* Neurophysiological support for the diagnosis of motor neuron disease relies on demonstrating widespread EMG denervation, indicating widespread anterior horn cell disease. It is usually important to examine muscles supplied by anterior horn cells in each of the four spinal regions:

a. *Bulbar*: tongue, facial muscles

b. *Cervical*: upper limbs

c. *Thoracic*: paraspinals, rectus abdominus

d. *Lumbosacral*: lower limbs.

Within each region the electromyographer ideally looks for evidence of denervation in muscles supplied by different peripheral nerves and different motor roots to show the process is diffuse, and to limit the chance of misinterpretation because of coexisting pathology, particularly radiculopathies since they are common in this patient population.

4. *Multifocal motor neuropathy* is a relatively rare, but treatable condition that can mimic motor neuron disease. Classically there is asymmetrical distal upper limb weakness without sensory loss or muscle wasting. Conduction block is suspected by the neurophysiologist when a muscle is weak, but not wasted, and has a normal CMAP following distal stimulation, provided the clinical context is appropriate. This latter point is essential, since, for example, patients with a stroke or myasthenia gravis will commonly have weak muscles that are not wasted and have normal CMAPs, but the explanation is not peripheral nerve conduction block.

To maximize the chance of proving motor conduction block the electrophysiologist should test clinically weak muscles. Conduction block can be very proximal, even in the motor roots, so cervical root stimulation may be helpful if there is no demonstrable block with standard more distal studies, but this is uncomfortable, so its use is generally limited. EMG of the weak muscle will often help distinguish conduction block from axon loss, but secondary axon loss in blocked nerves may make that distinction difficult. If nerve conduction studies appear to show conduction block in nerves supplying strong muscles the finding should be questioned, and submaximal proximal stimulation or anomalous innervation should be suspected. EMG of the muscle should help disprove motor conduction block.

5. *Detection of conduction block depends on the nerve studied.* Because of anatomical considerations it is easier, and more reliable, to demonstrate conduction block in some nerves than others. For example, the high stimulus intensity required to stimulate nerves supramaximally at Erb's point frequently results in activation of neighbouring areas of the brachial plexus. If recording median nerve conduction to the abductor pollicis brevis, the unwanted activation of axons destined for other muscles of the thenar eminence via the ulnar nerve can contaminate the CMAP, thereby reducing the ability to detect proximal median nerve conduction block. This problem is not incurred when testing for proximal block in ulnar nerve fibres to abductor digiti minimi, since axons in the median nerve activated by proximal stimulation do not innervate muscles particularly close to the abductor digiti minimi in the hypothenar eminence. In the lower limbs it may be difficult to prove conduction block because it can be difficult to ensure supramaximal

proximal stimulation, plus temporal dispersion can be quite marked because of the length of the nerves.

Role of nerve conduction/EMG in the diagnosis of motor neuron disease

- Confirm there is evidence of denervation consistent with anterior horn cell disease, not simply benign fasciculations.
- Rule out significant peripheral nerve pathology, such as multifocal motor neuropathy with conduction block, which may mimic upper limb presentations.
- Determine the extent of denervation in clinically unaffected areas, thus allowing a more confident early diagnosis, particularly with monomelic presentations.
- Follow up patients to look for spread of pathology over time, allowing an earlier and more confident diagnosis.

Limitations of nerve conduction/EMG in diagnosing motor neuron disease

- There may not be widespread denervation on EMG performed early in the course of motor neuron disease, so it may need to be repeated.
- Partial motor conduction block may be difficult to prove when it is very proximal.
- Multiple motor radiculopathies are common in the elderly, also causing denervation with normal sensory conduction.
- Widespread denervation alone does not necessarily imply motor neuron disease, but must be interpreted in light of the clinical presentation, presence of upper motor neuron signs, and other investigation results.

Case 2

Clinical presentation

A 41-year-old man is referred with an 11-month history of mild lower back pain with occasional shooting sensations radiating down the lateral aspect of his left leg. He has a garden on a steep incline, and over the past couple of weeks since referral he has noticed his left foot tends to slap down when he walks downhill.

He has mild weakness (MRC grade 4+) of left ankle dorsiflexion, inversion, and eversion. Plantar flexion is normal strength. Knee and ankle deep tendon reflexes are normal. There is poorly delineated subjective sensory disturbance over the dorsum of the foot and lower lateral calf. For results of nerve conduction studies and EMG see Tables 14.3 and 14.4.

Questions

1. Are there any neurophysiological clues to indicate whether the findings are new given the change in symptoms over the past couple of weeks?
2. Should paraspinal EMG have been performed?

Interpretation

The clinical presentation has progressed slightly since referral, and is very suggestive of a left L5 motor radiculopathy. The weakness of inversion argues against a peroneal neuropathy since tibialis posterior receives innervation via the tibial nerve. Similarly, the normal strength of plantar flexion, preserved ankle reflex, and normal sensation on the sole of the foot argues against a sciatic neuropathy or S1 radiculopathy. If it had been performed, a preserved soleus H-reflex would also suggest the S1 root is unaffected, but it adds no extra information in this context given the ankle reflex is preserved.

Nerve conduction studies show that sensory responses are normal, suggesting here that pathology is preganglionic. Remember that recording normal sensory responses implies that axonal pathology is likely to be preganglionic, but does not always imply that all pathology is preganglionic. For example, sensory responses remain normal with peripheral nerve demyelination proximal to both the recording and stimulating electrodes, and in disorders of the neuromuscular junction, or myopathies. In this case the normality of the left superficial peroneal sensory response is especially helpful since it carries L5 sensory fibres and helps rule out weakness due to postganglionic axonal lesions of the sciatic or peroneal nerves.

Table 14.3 Nerve conduction studies

Nerve	Stimulation	Recording	Amplitude (μV or mV)			Onset latency (ms)			Conduction velocity (m/s)			F wave latency (ms)		
			R	L	N	R	L	N	R	L	N	R	L	N
Sensory														
Sural	Calf	Posterior ankle	17	16	**≥10**				41	40	**≥40**			
Superficial peroneal	Lateral ankle	Dorsum of foot	8	9	**≥5**				40	44	**≥40**			
Motor														
Tibial	Ankle	AH	11.2	8.0	**≥4**	4.1	4.2	**≤5.8**						**≤56**
	Knee	AH	10.9	6.8					45	45	**≥41**			
Peroneal	Ankle	EDB	3.2	1.0	**≥2**	4.3	4.5	**≤6.5**						**≤56**
	Fibular head	EDB	3.0	1.0					42	44	**≥41**			
	Popliteal fossa	EDB	3.0	0.9					51	50				

Sensory amplitudes are μV, motor amplitudes mV. R, right; L, left; N, normal; AH, abductor hallucis brevis; EDB extensor digitorum brevis.

Table 14.4 EMG

Muscle	Spontaneous activity	Motor unit action potential			Recruitment	Interference pattern
		Duration	Amplitude	Phases		
L tibialis anterior	Nil	↑	↑	↑	Reduced	↓
L tibialis posterior	1+ fibs	↑↑	↑↑	↑	Reduced	↓↓
L peroneus longus	1+ fibs	↑	↑	↑	Reduced	↓
L vastus medialis	Nil	N	N	N	N	N
L medial gastrocnemius	Nil	N	N	N	Poor activation	↓
L gluteus maximus	Nil	N	N	N	N	N
L gluteus medius	Nil	↑	N	↑	Reduced	↓

↑, mildly increased; ↑↑, moderately increased; ↓, mildly decreased; ↓↓, moderately decreased; L, left; N, normal; fibs, fibrillation potentials.

The slightly small CMAP from the left extensor digitorum brevis probably reflects partial axon degeneration. In theory this may be due to pathology anywhere along the axon, but the normality of sensory responses suggests the site of damage is preganglionic. Caution has to be taken with interpretation of CMAPs from the extensor digitorum brevis muscle since it can be damaged by trivial local trauma not relevant to the clinical presentation.

EMG shows evidence of partial denervation in all muscles examined that receive L5 root innervation, irrespective of which peripheral nerve innervates them, although the apparent severity of findings is variable. There is no denervation in L3/4 innervated muscles (left vastus medialis) or in muscles receiving S1 root innervation (left medial gastrocnemius and gluteus maximus), thus localizing the pathology to the left L5 motor root.

The motor unit action potentials seen on EMG are both abnormally prolonged and high amplitude. Such changes take at least several weeks to develop, suggesting that some degree of remodelling of motor units predates the recent weakness noticed just a couple of weeks prior to EMG examination.

Conclusion

The neurophysiological examination is suggestive of a left L5 radiculopathy. There is no evidence of a peroneal or sciatic neuropathy.

Comment: neurophysiological assessment of radiculopathies

1. *Patchy EMG findings.* EMG findings in radiculopathies can be patchy, with some muscles supplied by the affected root seemingly more denervated than others. There are a number of potential reasons for this other than missing pathology due to patchy EMG sampling. Firstly, the pathology may only affect some fascicles of the root, leaving others relatively unaffected. Secondly, the root innervation of a muscle may vary slightly from one subject to another, either with different weightings of innervation by the usual roots, or even completely different root supplies. There is some evidence for this in infants, in whom deltoid function may recover due to C7 innervation despite complete avulsion of the C5 and C6 motor roots during birth. To some extent the variation in myotomes noted between different textbooks depends on how they were determined—cadaveric anatomy versus neurosurgical or EMG evidence. Finally, the timing of EMG examination with respect to injury will affect the amount of spontaneous EMG activity expected in different muscles innervated by the same root since proximal muscles, such as paraspinals or glutei, can develop fibrillation potentials within a week or so, long before distal muscles, but they will also be the first muscles to show recovery with reinnervation.

2. *Paraspinal EMG* can be very helpful in localization of axonal pathology, since denervation should only occur with lesions proximal to the dorsal ramus, either at motor root level or affecting the cell body of the motor neuron. In practice, similar information is often gained by demonstrating that sensory potentials are normal, implying that axonal pathology is preganglionic. However, if sensory responses are absent due to a coexisting neuropathy, or unobtainable for another reason such as peripheral oedema, paraspinal EMG can help. Furthermore, in the setting of recent nerve root trauma a week or two prior to examination, the proximal location of the paraspinal muscles means they will be the first, and potentially only, muscles to show fibrillation potentials on EMG.

However, there are limitations to interpreting paraspinal EMG. First, any abnormality is relatively poorly localized in the rostro-caudal axis since paraspinal muscles receive innervation from several overlapping spinal roots. Second, if there has been previous spinal surgery the finding of spontaneous fibrillation potentials has little or no significance. Third, the normal morphology of paraspinal muscle motor unit action potentials is relatively spiky, and they are difficult to recruit smoothly or fully, making the interpretation of activity other than spontaneous activity difficult. Finally, in radiculopathies where there is a degree of recovery, fibrillations and positive sharp waves will disappear first from the paraspinals, in which case paraspinal EMG may be normal.

3. *Sensory responses in radiculopathies.* In radiculopathies the sensory response amplitudes are characteristically normal since the dorsal root ganglion lies distal to the lesion. It can be helpful to compare sensory responses from the affected side to the unaffected, even if they appear normal. For example, a sural response of 15μV is generally considered within normal limits, but if the amplitude from the unaffected side is 45μV it suggests it is probably pathologically reduced. Occasionally it may be possible to have reduced sensory amplitudes secondary to lumbosacral radiculopathy since, in this region, it has been documented that the dorsal root ganglion can lie very proximal, even within the spinal canal.

4. *Motor responses in radiculopathies.* CMAP amplitude is a relatively insensitive marker of motor root pathology since muscles usually receive innervation from two or more roots, with variable weightings. Even complete loss of one motor root will have an unpredictable effect on the relevant CMAP amplitude, which may be affected very little. Thus, in contrast to mononeuropathies or axonal polyneuropathies, loss of CMAP amplitude is generally less helpful in quantifying axon loss in radiculopathies. F-waves are also of limited use in the investigation of radiculopathies for similar reasons—a

normal F-wave response may be maintained if just one of the roots to that muscle is functioning normally.

5. *Lumbosacral radiculopathies versus plexopathies.* The neurophysiological assessment of lumbosacral radiculopathies and plexopathies is generally less satisfactory than upper limb examination for a number of reasons. First, there are fewer readily recorded sensory nerves in the lower limbs with which to prove whether axonal pathology is pre or postganglionic. These may be impossible to record if there is peripheral oedema, and even without oedema the absence of superficial peroneal (predominantly L5) or saphenous (mainly L4) sensory responses is not necessarily helpful in localizing pathology, especially in elderly patients, as they may be damaged by trivial local trauma. Second, paraspinal EMG may not help since fibrillations are lost first with early reinnervation, and even if found they are not specific to a particular root level because of overlapping innervation. Third, muscles studied with routine needle EMG receive little if any innervation from the S2 roots or lower, making this region of the spine invisible to routine neurophysiological studies. Finally, interpretation is further confounded by the observation that the dorsal root ganglion may occasionally lie within the spinal canal in the lower lumbosacral region. In this case, sensory responses could be absent due to central spine or root pathology which would normally be considered 'preganglionic'. All these factors mean it can be difficult to determine exactly which lumbosacral root is affected, and in some cases it may even be difficult to distinguish a radiculopathy from a plexopathy, especially in elderly patients with oedema.

6. *Nerve root versus disc level.* The spinal cord terminates to become the cauda equina in the upper lumbar region (see Fig. 14.1). This means that disc disease in the lumbosacral region may cause nerve root pathology at the level expected, or may affect lower roots. For example, the L4/5 disc may conceivably herniate laterally to affect the L4 root, or more likely the L5 root. With a large posterior herniation several roots may be affected bilaterally: cauda equina syndrome. This does not happen in the higher cervical and thoracic cord, although occasionally roots may exit the spinal canal a level above or below that expected. EMG examination, of course, tells us about the nerve root affected, and not the disc.

7. *EMG may remain normal in a radiculopathy*, particularly when there is no demonstrable weakness or loss of tendon reflex. Although this can relate to mild pathology and EMG sampling error, it may also occur when there is nerve root demyelination without axon loss, or when the dorsal (sensory) root is affected in isolation, thereby leaving the motor axons unaffected. EMG therefore cannot rule out a radiculopathy, but complements MRI.

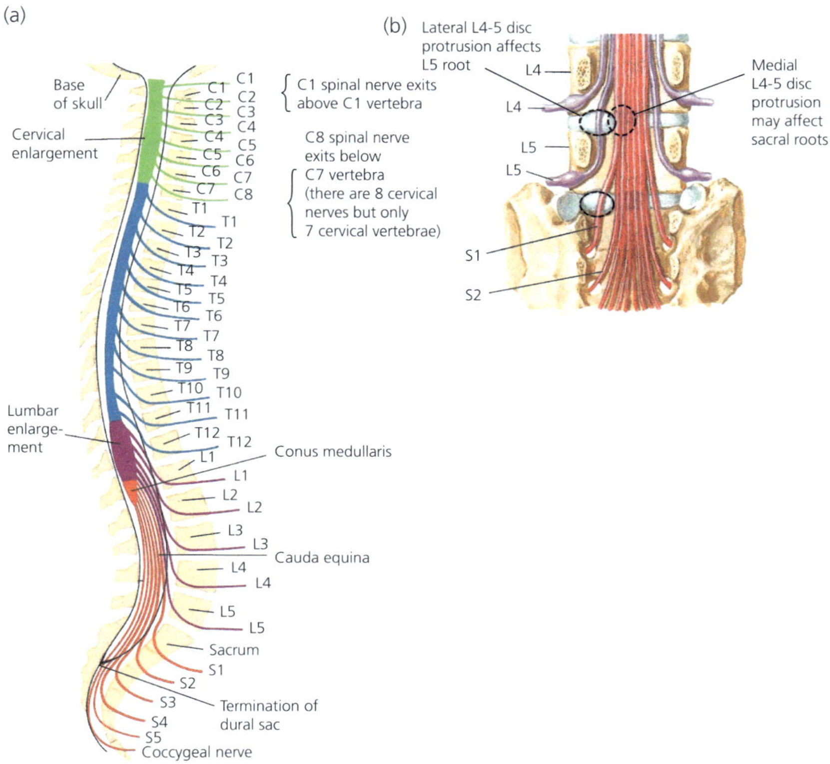

Figure 14.1 (a) Spine with exit level of all roots, and (b) lumbosacral spine with site of roots exiting in relation to disc pathology.

Role of nerve conduction/EMG studies in radiculopathies

- Rule out entrapment neuropathies and other mimicking conditions.
- Determine the most likely spinal root(s) involved—especially if multilevel degenerative disease is seen on MRI and clinical assessment is challenging.
- Help confirm that a lesion seen on MRI is causing axon loss, thus supporting clinical suspicion that it is likely to be causing radicular symptoms.
- Occasionally help confirm a radioculopathy when MRI is negative.
- EMG can sometimes help indicate the age and severity of pathology, although neither can be assessed very accurately.

Limitations of nerve conduction/EMG studies in radiculopathies

- EMG cannot exclude a radiculopathy since it relies on loss of motor axons. If there is demyelination, or if the dorsal root is selectively affected, there will be no EMG or nerve conduction abnormality.
- In the lumbosacral region posterior disc herniation may impinge on a root lower than expected, so EMG findings may appear not to correspond to the level of the diseased disc.
- It can be hard to distinguish a lumbosacral plexopathy from a radiculopathy if distal sensory responses are unrecordable, and given the limitations of paraspinal EMG.
- The lower sacral roots are not examined by routine EMG.

Case 3

Clinical presentation

A 34-year-old woman developed severe pain around her neck and right upper scapular region whilst in hospital for surgery to a traumatically fractured femur. She was given analgesia for the pain, which slowly eased over several days, and mild shoulder weakness was not investigated. Now 6 weeks later she has mild weakness (MRC grade 4+) of right deltoid, supraspinatus, and infraspinatus, and some rather ill-defined sensory loss overlying a small area of the right deltoid and lateral forearm. There is also very mild weakness of flexion of the distal phalanx of the right thumb. For results of nerve conduction studies and EMG see Tables 14.5 and 14.6.

Questions

1. What would the EMG have shown in the first few days whilst she had the pain?
2. What do you make of the EMG findings in the flexor pollicis longus?

Interpretation

The sensory response recorded from the right superficial radial nerve is about 40% smaller than that on the left, but this is weak evidence of pathology since it lies within the normal range, and a side-to-side amplitude difference of about 50% is commonly accepted as significant given biological variation and the reproducibility of sensory amplitudes. The response from the right lateral cutaneous nerve of the forearm is rather more convincingly reduced, providing more robust confirmation of partial axon loss, albeit from a nerve that can sometimes be harder to record.

Motor conduction studies remain largely normal, but the median and ulnar motor conduction studies test axons to the abductor pollicis brevis and abductor digiti minimi muscles respectively. These pass via the lower trunk of the brachial plexus, and the C8/T1 roots, and are not clinically affected, so would be expected to remain normal. Although the CMAP from the right deltoid is smaller than the left this degree of difference is not a very robust finding, so is of questionable significance without needle EMG, which provides a more sensitive test of motor axon loss.

Clinically it seems probable that sensory loss over the deltoid is in the cutaneous distribution of the axillary nerve, which would fit with the EMG evidence of partial denervation of the right deltoid, and imply an axillary

Table 14.5 Nerve conduction studies

Nerve	Stimulation	Recording	Amplitude (μV or mV)			Onset latency (ms)			Conduction velocity (m/s)			F wave latency (ms)		
			R	L	N	R	L	N	R	L	N	R	L	N
Sensory														
Median	Index finger	Wrist	12	13	**≥7**			**≤3.5**	53	52	**≥49**			
	Middle finger	Wrist	16	16	**≥7**			**≤3.5**	54	55	**≥49**			
Ulnar	Little finger	Wrist	11	7	**≥5**			**≤3.1**	53	50	**≥49**			
Radial	Forearm	Snuff box	31	52	**≥12**			**≤3.0**	58	63	**≥50**			
Medial cut n of forearm	Medial elbow	Medial forearm	6	7	**≥5**			**≤2.5**	53	53	**≥50**			
Lateral cut n of forearm	Antecubital fossa	Lateral elbow	4	12	**≥8**			**≤2.5**	50	54	**≥50**			
Motor														
Median	Wrist	APB	8.9	8.1	**≥4**	3.4	3.4	**≤4.2**				28	29	**≤31**
	Elbow	APB	8.5	8.0					54	51	**≥49**			
Ulnar	Wrist	ADM	9.8		**≥6**	2.7		**≤3.3**				30		**≤32**
	Below elbow	ADM	9.9						56		**≥49**			
	Above elbow	ADM	9.7						50					
	Axilla	ADM	9.5						58					
Axillary	Erb's point	Deltoid	2.9	4.9	**≥3**	3.9	3.8	**≤4.9**						

Sensory amplitudes are μV, motor amplitudes mV. cut n, cutaneous nerve; R, right; L, left; N, normal; APB, abductor pollicis brevis; ADM, abductor digiti minimi.

Table 14.6 EMG

Muscle	Spontaneous activity	Motor unit action potential			Recruitment	Interference pattern
		Duration	Amplitude	Phases		
R 1st dorsal interosseous	Nil	N	N	N	N	N
R abductor pollicis brevis	Nil	N	N	N	N	N
R abductor digiti minimi	Nil	N	N	N	N	N
R flexor pollicis longus	Nil	N	N	↑	Reduced	↓
R extensor digitorum communis	Nil	N	N	N	N	N
R triceps	Nil	N	N	N	N	N
R biceps	Nil	N	N	N	N	N
R deltoid	2+ fibs	↑	N	↑	Reduced	↓↓
L deltoid	Nil	N	N	N	N	N
R infraspinatus	1+ fibs	↑	N	↑	Reduced	↓
R serratus anterior	Nil	N	N	N	N	N

↑, mildly increased; ↓, mildly decreased; ↓↓, moderately decreased; R, right; L, left; N, normal; fibs, fibrillation potentials.

neuropathy. There is also evidence of partial denervation of infraspinatus, suggesting axon loss in the suprascapular nerve. Although clinically affected, the supraspinatus was not examined by the electromyographer since it is supplied by the same nerve. Finally, EMG suggests mild denervation of flexor pollicis longus, which in the context of normal EMG of abductor pollicis brevis, suggests axon loss in the anterior interosseous nerve, but not the main trunk of the median nerve.

EMG of weak muscles shows a mild increase in motor unit action potential polyphasia and duration, but not amplitude. The changes are mild, and compatible with subacute axonal pathology, in this case of about 6 weeks' duration, in which there has been time for motor unit remodelling to start. Compare this to chronic severe, yet stable, neurogenic conditions where motor unit action potentials tend to be very broad and high amplitude but not especially polyphasic, and where spontaneous EMG activity may disappear. Despite the relatively mild changes in motor unit action potential morphology the associated fibrillation potentials, reduced recruitment and interference pattern confirm the suspicion of partial denervation.

If the EMG had been performed acutely, within the first few days of experiencing severe neck and shoulder pain, there would not have been time for Wallerian degeneration of the axons or motor unit remodelling. On EMG there would not have been fibrillation potentials, and the motor unit action potentials would still have normal morphology. Motor unit recruitment would have been abnormal for two reasons. Firstly, pain is likely to have had a dominant effect early on, resulting in poor activation of the muscle. Secondly, the degeneration of axons, albeit relatively mild and not yet complete, would result in a reduced pool of functional motor units and therefore reduced recruitment when the muscle is contracted—resulting in a tendency for motor units to fire at high rates in relative isolation. The EMG performed this early would provide limited information, and because of the time course of Wallerian degeneration there would not yet be changes in sensory or motor conduction studies. A repeat study would be necessary.

Conclusion

There is neurophysiological evidence of partial axon loss in the right axillary, suprascapular, anterior interosseous, and lateral forearm cutaneous nerves. In this context it supports the clinical suspicion of brachial neuritis (neuralgic amyotrophy).

Comment: neurophysiological assessment of brachial plexopathies

1. *Motor conduction to proximal muscles.* In the case presented here most electromyographers would choose not to measure motor conduction to the weak supraspinatus and infraspinatus muscles. It is possible to stimulate the suprascapular nerve and measure a CMAP from these muscles, but this technique cannot detect axonal pathology as sensitively as needle EMG, and the CMAP is not as reproducible as it is from smaller distal upper limb muscles. This is in part because of variability of recording electrode placement. Here, as in many clinical contexts, enough information can be obtained to make a diagnosis even though these muscles are examined by needle EMG alone. There are still occasions when it can be very helpful to record proximal muscle CMAPs, for example, if there is clinical suspicion of demyelination that cannot be proven elsewhere a prolonged distal motor latency would be informative.

2. *Nerve involvement in brachial neuritis.* It is common for brachial neuritis to result in patchy loss of axons, particularly affecting the suprascapular, axillary, long thoracic, and anterior interosseous nerves. Thus the upper aspects of the brachial plexus and its branches are more susceptible than the lower portions, often resulting in weakness around the shoulder. To help distinguish preganglionic from postganglionic pathology it is therefore useful to check sensory responses from nerves carrying C5 and C6 fibres that pass through the upper plexus: the lateral cutaneous nerve of the forearm, median sensory response from the thumb or index finger, and the superficial radial nerve. In textbook brachial neuritis, some of these sensory response amplitudes may be reduced, helping to confirm axonal pathology distal to the dorsal root ganglion. However, the sensory responses not infrequently remain entirely normal in brachial neuritis, presumably showing the patchy nature of the pathology, or involvement of nerves after they have left the plexus, rather than the plexus itself. When sensory responses are entirely normal the neurophysiology only shows patchy motor axon loss, therefore may be compatible with motor root or anterior horn cell pathology. The history generally helps make the distinction, but paraspinal EMG may be of some help too in detecting pathology proximal to the dorsal ramus (resulting in fibrillations), however this distinction is not absolute.

3. *Thoracic outlet syndrome and assessment of the lower brachial plexus.* Neurophysiological examination is an excellent way of testing the lower portions of the brachial plexus, and distinguishing, for example, an ulnar neuropathy, C8/T1 radiculopathy and a lower trunk brachial plexopathy. A common request is to examine for evidence of suspected neurogenic thoracic outlet

syndrome, although the frequency of confirming this syndrome tends to be low. In this condition axonal damage to the lower trunk can result in reduced or absent sensory responses from the little finger (ulnar nerve) and the medial cutaneous nerve of the forearm. Nerve conduction and EMG confirm loss of motor axons to muscles innervated by axons traversing the lower trunk and C8/T1 roots, especially the abductor pollicis brevis, but also the abductor digiti minimi and first dorsal interosseous muscles. From a neurophysiological perspective, lower trunk pathology is generally easy to distinguish from an ulnar neuropathy since the latter would not affect median nerve innervated muscles and focal slowing can generally be demonstrated. C8 or T1 radiculopathies would not result in abnormal sensory responses since the pathology is preganglionic.

4. *Plexopathies following radiotherapy.* Patients sometimes present with progressive weakness many years after intensive radiotherapy to tissue in close proximity to the brachial plexus. The classic EMG finding in radiotherapy-induced plexopathies is neurogenic change with myokymia and fasciculations, implying spontaneous discharges of the motor axon. However, it is not specific, and not always present, and usually the gradual progression of weakness without pain helps distinguish radiation-related damage from tumour infiltration, which tends to be painful and more rapidly progressive. Another clue can be that late radiation damage often preferentially affects the upper portions of the brachial plexus, whereas tumour infiltration frequently affects the lower portions. Proximal conduction block has been reported in radiotherapy-induced plexopathies, which can even result in difficulty in discriminating this from inflammatory demyelinating neuropathies depending on the wider clinical presentation.

5. *Lumbosacral plexopathies.* It may be difficult to distinguish lumbosacral plexopathies from radiculopathies for a number of reasons. There are not reliable, routine sensory conduction studies to separate pre- from postganglionic axonal pathology affecting the mid/upper lumbar plexus or the lower sacral plexus. Even commonly recorded sural (mainly S1) and superficial peroneal (mainly L5) sensory responses may be absent in the elderly or due to peripheral oedema. Paraspinal EMG may well provide little additional information, particularly in the elderly, and routine lower limb EMG studies do not examine the lower sacral roots.

Role of nerve conduction/EMG studies in plexopathies

- Rule out entrapment neuropathies, radiculopathies, and other mimicking conditions.
- Assess the distribution of pathology within the plexus since this may not be clinically apparent, especially if examination is limited by pain.
- Gauge the severity of pathology, and help determine prognosis.
- In traumatic plexopathies the distinction of nerve root avulsion (pre-gangionic) from plexus pathology can help guide management and prognosis.
- Myokymia on EMG may provide a clue to aetiology when weakness develops years after radiotherapy, but it is not specific.

Limitations of nerve conduction/EMG studies in plexopathies

- If pathology is demyelination rather than axon loss it may not be detected since distal sensory and motor responses will remain normal, and there will be no denervation on EMG.
- Localization of pathology in the lumbosacral plexus may be difficult due to limited sensory conduction studies beyond L4, L5, and S1, and limited EMG (lower sacral roots not examined).
- If peripheral sensory responses are unobtainable, for example, due to oedema, it may be difficult to distinguish plexopathies from radiculopathies (paraspinal EMG may help).
- Plexopathies can be patchy, and it may not be possible to localize pathology precisely.

Case 4

Clinical presentation

A 42-year-old taxi driver was referred because of numbness of the little and ring fingers of his right hand. He had become particularly aware of this over the preceding 8 weeks, but in retrospect felt the sensation had not been quite right for almost a year. Examination revealed mild weakness (MRC grade 4) and wasting of his abductor digiti minimi and first dorsal interosseous muscles, with no weakness in radial or median nerve territories, and normal strength in the ulnar innervated portion of flexor digitorum profundus. Sensory loss involved the palmar and dorsal surfaces of the ulnar border of his right hand, including the little and ring fingers. There was no objective sensory loss proximal to the wrist. For results of nerve conduction studies and EMG see Tables 14.7 and 14.8.

Questions

1. What is the prognosis for recovery?
2. Has a C8 radiculopathy been excluded?

Interpretation

The right ulnar sensory response is absent, implying that there is postganglionic axon loss affecting the ulnar nerve, but this result alone does not localize the pathology. However, the finding of conduction slowing and partial motor conduction block at the elbow does locate the site of pathology. This could probably have been localized further by short segment studies, in which the stimulating electrode is moved by measured increments along the nerve around the elbow, starting distally, to find the position at which there is a sudden change in CMAP amplitude and latency, implying the pathology (partial conduction block) is between that stimulation site and the previous one.

Note that if there was pure conduction block at the elbow without axon loss, the distal axon would remain functional, and there would be no reduction in ulnar sensory response from the little finger since both the stimulation and recording sites are distal to the lesion. In this case, however, the unilateral loss of ulnar sensory response suggests there is sensory axon loss. This is further confirmed by the asymmetry of CMAP amplitudes from the left versus right abductor digiti minimi in response to distal stimulation, and the EMG findings, both demonstrating motor axon loss. Clinically both partial motor conduction block and axon loss contribute to weakness, but only the latter causes wasting.

Table 14.7 Nerve conduction studies

Nerve	Stimulation	Recording	Amplitude (μV or mV)			Onset latency (ms)			Conduction velocity (m/s)			F wave latency (ms)		
			R	L	N	R	L	N	R	L	N	R	L	N
Sensory														
Median	Middle finger	Wrist	13		**≥7**			**≤3.5**	56		**≥49**			
Ulnar	Little finger	Wrist	Absent	7	**≥5**			**≤3.1**		55	**≥49**			
Ulnar	Wrist	Elbow	Absent		**≥20**						**≥50**			
Radial	Forearm	Snuff box	33		**≥12**			**≤3.0**	62		**≥50**			
Motor														
Median	Wrist	APB	8.8		**≥4**	3.5		**≤4.2**						**≤31**
	Elbow	APB	8.8						55		**≥49**			
Ulnar	Wrist	ADM	5.4	11.0	**≥6**	3.1	3.1	**≤3.3**						**≤32**
	Below elbow	ADM	5.0	10.8					54	57	**≥49**			
	Above elbow	ADM	2.1	10.2					32	56	**≥49**			
	Erb's	ADM	2.0						49		**≥49**			

Sensory amplitudes are μV, motor amplitudes mV. R, right; L, left; N, normal; APB, abductor pollicis brevis; ADM, abductor digiti minimi.

Table 14.8 EMG

Muscle	Spontaneous activity	Motor unit action potential			Recruitment	Interference pattern
		Duration	Amplitude	Phases		
R 1st dorsal interosseous	2+ fibs, fascics	↑	↑↑	↑↑	Reduced	↓↓
R flexor carpi ulnaris	Nil	N	↑	↑	Mildly reduced	↓
R extensor digitorum communis	Nil	N	N	N	N	N
R flexor pollicis longus	Nil	N	N	N	N	N

↑, mildly increased; ↑↑, moderately increased; ↓, mildly decreased; ↓↓, moderately decreased; R, right; N, normal; fascics, fasciculation potentials; fibs, fibrillation potentials.

EMG shows evidence of partial denervation of muscles innervated by the ulnar nerve, with the first dorsal interosseous more affected than the flexor carpi ulnaris. This is a common finding, and probably reflects variation in the susceptibility of the different fascicles of the ulnar nerve at the elbow, although inadequate sampling is always a potential confounder. On EMG a slight reduction in the recruitment of motor units due to conduction block will be almost impossible to detect here because axon loss also reduces recruitment. The preferential involvement of different fascicles is sometimes investigated by performing ulnar motor conduction to the first dorsal interosseous in addition the abductor digiti minimi.

There are many factors arguing against the possibility of a C8 radiculopathy. This is unlikely from the clinical presentation of sensory loss in a typical ulnar distribution plus weakness limited to ulnar innervated muscles. From a neurophysiological perspective the absence of right ulnar sensory response suggests there is postganglionic axon loss, therefore arguing against a radiculopathy. Finally, muscles receiving innervation from axons traversing the C8 root but not subsequently travelling in the ulnar nerve are unaffected: the extensor digitorum communis (radial nerve) and the flexor pollicis longus (median nerve).

In this case the history revealed a clue to the likely aetiology, since the patient tended to drive with his right elbow resting on the door of his right-hand drive car, and this would exacerbate his symptoms. Provided the patient modifies his behaviour and protects his elbow the conduction block may well recover in 1–3 months. Axon loss, on the other hand, takes longer to recover since axons regrow at approximately 1–2mm/day. In the meantime, distal remodelling of motor units provides some ongoing compensation for the loss of motor axons, and is reflected in the abnormal EMG.

Conclusion

There is evidence of a right ulnar neuropathy at the elbow, with partial motor conduction block plus evidence of sensory and motor axon loss. There is no evidence of a cervical radiculopathy.

Comment: neurophysiological assessment of focal neuropathies

1. *Confirming conduction block*. The finding of conduction block is very important in this case as it helps localize the lesion and provides a more favourable prognosis for rapid recovery than severe axonal injury in isolation. If conduction block is found, the neurophysiologist should first increase the proximal

stimulus intensity to ensure it is not simply a technical error reflecting insufficient depolarization. Where possible it is helpful to stimulate at an additional site proximal to the suspected block to provide reassurance that the finding is true – the CMAP should remain similar with the second site of stimulation proximal to the block. Clinically, muscles innervated by nerves with motor conduction block should be weak corresponding to the amount of block. If there is no axon loss they will not be wasted, whereas with axon loss the muscle will be wasted provided sufficient time has elapsed.

2. *Criteria for conduction block.* There are a number of published criteria that help define whether conduction block is definite or probable, initially developed for research studies. There are three main issues to consider. First, when the distal CMAP is small it may be impossible to be certain that a further decrease with proximal stimulation is due to conduction block rather than an artefact or other non-significant finding. Second, a problem arises when there is temporal dispersion of the CMAP elicited by proximal stimulation. This is common and results in a CMAP that is low in amplitude, just like conduction block, but with much longer duration. With temporal dispersion there is little loss in CMAP area, unlike conduction block, and the pathological implication is quite different, temporal dispersion suggesting a patchy process causing variable degrees of conduction slowing in different axons. There are therefore upper limits to the amount of temporal dispersion allowed when making a diagnosis of definite or probable conduction block. Third, conduction block is more reliably diagnosed in some nerves than others. To some extent this reflects the difficulty in ensuring supramaximal proximal stimulation of some nerves, for example, a significant percentage reduction in CMAP amplitude in the ulnar nerve may not be significant in the tibial nerve. In addition, block is difficult to detect if high intensity proximal stimulation tends to activate neighbouring nerves whose muscles might contaminate the CMAP because of their proximity to the muscle being recorded.

3. *Sensory conduction is affected first in mild compressive neuropathies.* In the case presented here sensory responses are absent whilst motor responses remain recordable. This is relatively common in compressive focal neuropathies, such as carpal tunnel syndrome or ulnar neuropathies at the elbow. In general, the first and only abnormality detected in very mild focal neuropathies is slowing of sensory conduction. Clearly this is better detected in carpal tunnel syndrome, where stimulation and recording sites are on opposite sides of the lesion, than ulnar neuropathies at the elbow where the pathology is proximal to the usual sensory nerve stimulation and recording sites (see point 5). In moderate severity lesions there is usually a clear reduction in amplitude or complete loss of sensory response, often with relatively normal or only mildly

reduced CMAP amplitude but evidence of slowing of motor conduction or partial conduction block across the site of compression. Finally, only in severe lesions is slowing of motor conduction accompanied by marked motor axon loss and a reduction in CMAP amplitude even with distal stimulation.

4. *Fascicular injury.* Nerves are arranged in fascicles, thus it is not surprising that these can be affected differently when a nerve is injured. Indeed this is a fairly common finding in mononeuropathies, and in the case presented here the flexor carpi ulnaris appears to be less severely denervated than the first dorsal interosseous muscle, possibly because of the different susceptibilities of their respective fascicles. This is obviously important to know when framing a differential diagnosis, and when gauging severity of injury. Another common example of differential nerve injury occurs following a stretch/compression injury to the sciatic nerve during hip operations. This often affects the peroneal division with relative sparing of tibial fibres even though the site of injury is proximal, at a point where the two divisions run together. This probably reflects the susceptibility of peroneal nerve axons due to their position lateral to tibial fibres, plus the relatively tight tethering of the peroneal nerve at both its proximal end and distally at the fibular head, rendering it more susceptible to stretch damage. The microarchitecture of the peroneal nerve axons and their blood supply also probably plays a role.

5. *Sensory conduction block in the ulnar nerve at the elbow* will generally pass undetected by routine sensory conduction tests since the distal axon remains functional, and since both stimulation and recording sites are distal to the site of block. If there is minimal motor block this may remain below the detection threshold of conduction studies. In theory mixed nerve tests, stimulating both sensory and motor fibres at the wrist and recording them at the elbow, might detect partial sensory block but they are not always performed, and are not sensitive to mild sensory conduction block. Thus the patient with sensory abnormalities in a convincing ulnar distribution but no weakness (implying no significant motor conduction block or axon loss) might have a normal neurophysiological examination despite partial sensory conduction block. Of course, the same presentation caused by sensory axon loss would generally be detected because of reduced sensory response amplitudes.

6. *Ulnar neuropathies at the wrist* are far less common than at the elbow. The neurophysiological principles of localization and assessment of severity are comparable to those for any focal neuropathy, and require knowledge of the local anatomy. Motor conduction is performed to the first dorsal interosseous as well as the abductor digiti minimi to test the deep palmar branch of the nerve, looking for conduction delay (prolonged distal motor latency) or CMAP amplitude reduction. The pattern of neurophysiological findings

depends on the exact site and severity of the lesion. Demonstration that the dorsal ulnar cutaneous branch is unaffected provides some additional support for a distal lesion, but it can remain unaffected in fascicular lesions at the elbow, so it should not be over interpreted in isolation.

Role of nerve conduction/EMG studies in ulnar neuropathies

- Localize the lesion, the elbow being a more common site than Guyon's canal at the wrist.
- Rule out a C8 radiculopathy, lower trunk brachial plexopathy, and other mimicking conditions.
- Gauge the severity of pathology, and the contribution of axon loss versus conduction block to help predict prognosis and guide treatment.
- The ulnar nerve can be stimulated right along its course to root level, so it is usually possible to demonstrate even relatively proximal motor conduction block.

Limitations of nerve conduction/EMG studies in ulnar neuropathies

- A significant proportion of patients with short duration symptoms experience spontaneous resolution, particularly with demyelinating pathology. There is a need to improve the evidence base for planning surgery on the basis of neurophysiological tests.
- Conduction block predominantly affecting sensory fibres at the elbow may pass undetected on neurophysiological examination (the patient has sensory symptoms only, no weakness).
- Fascicular pathology can, for example, mean that motor conduction to the abductor digiti minimi remains normal, but it is abnormal to the first dorsal interosseous. This should be suspected if there is differential weakness on clinical examination—it is important to test weak muscles.
- A normal response from the dorsal ulnar cutaneous nerve does not imply that the ulnar neuropathy must be at the wrist—it can remain normal in fascicular lesions at the elbow.

Case 5

Clinical presentation

A 76-year-old semi-retired farmer presents with wrist pain and numbness in the right hand. When questioned directly he reports that this has been the case for at least a couple of years, which he attributes to an old wrist fracture, but he also experiences a rather non-specific reduction in sensation from the toes of both feet. He was diagnosed with type II diabetes 3 years previously. Examination reveals marked wasting of the right thenar eminence, with weakness of the abductor pollicis brevis, but other small muscles of the hand are normal power, as is flexor pollicis longus. Ankle reflexes are absent, but other deep tendon reflexes are preserved. There is poorly defined loss of sensation maximal over the radial side of the right hand. For results of nerve conduction studies and EMG see Tables 14.9 and 14.10.

Questions

1. Why has median conduction to the second lumbrical been measured, and has this helped localize the site of pathology?
2. Is there a generalized neuropathy?

Interpretation

The lack of sural sensory response and small ulnar sensory response are not surprising in a manual worker of this age, and do not provide strong evidence of pathology. However, the absence of median nerve sensory response is abnormal since it would normally be slightly greater amplitude than the ulnar response. The pathology affecting median sensory fibres could, in theory at least, be either axon loss or conduction block between the stimulating and recording electrodes, for example, at the carpal tunnel.

The absence of a recordable CMAP from the right abductor pollicis brevis is in keeping with severe axon loss in the median nerve, although in theory conduction block distal to the site of stimulation could also result in a reduced or absent CMAP. This latter possibility does not fit here given the severe muscle wasting. However, because there is no response there is no evidence of conduction slowing, therefore neither routine sensory nor motor conduction studies can localize the site of pathology along the median nerve.

The second lumbrical/interosseous study is particularly helpful here since there is a CMAP obtainable from the second lumbrical following median nerve stimulation. The distal motor latency is very prolonged compared to the comparable ulnar nerve study to the interosseous muscle recorded by the

Table 14.9 Nerve conduction studies

Nerve	Stimulation	Recording	Amplitude (μV or mV)			Onset latency (ms)			Conduction velocity (m/s)			F wave latency (ms)		
			R	L	N	R	L	N	R	L	N	R	L	N
Sensory														
Median	Index finger	Wrist	Absent		**≥7**			**≤3.5**			**≥49**			
	Middle finger	Wrist	Absent		**≥7**			**≤3.5**			**≥49**			
Ulnar	Little finger	Wrist	3.2		**≥5**			**≤3.1**	48		**≥49**			
Radial	Forearm	Snuff box	15.7		**≥12**			**≤3.0**	54		**≥50**			
Sural	Calf	Posterior ankle	Absent		**≥10**			**≤3.8**			**≥40**			
Superficial peroneal	Lateral ankle	Dorsum of foot	Absent		**≥5**			**≤3.8**			**≥40**			
Motor														
Median	Wrist	APB	Absent		**≥4**			**≤4.2**						**≤31**
	Elbow	APB	Absent								**≥49**			
Ulnar	Wrist	ADM	7.1		**≥6**	3.1		**≤3.3**						**≤32**
	Below elbow	ADM	6.5						48		**≥49**			
	Above elbow	ADM	6.2						43		**≥49**			
Median	Wrist	2nd lumbrical	0.3			10.7		**≤4.0**						**≤56**
	Elbow	2nd lumbrical	0.3						39		**≥49**			
Ulnar	Wrist	Interosseous	3.2			3.4		**≤3.5**						
Peroneal	Ankle	EDB	2.1		**≥2**	5.8		**≤6.5**						**≤56**
	Fibular head	EDB	1.9						39		**≥41**			

Sensory amplitudes are μV, motor amplitudes mV. R, right; L, left; N, normal; APB, abductor pollicis brevis; ADM, abductor digiti minimi; EDB, extensor digitorum brevis.

Table 14.10 EMG

Muscle	Spontaneous activity	Motor unit action potential			Recruitment	Interference pattern
		Duration	Amplitude	Phases		
R 1st dorsal interosseous	Nil	N	N	N	N	N
R abductor pollicis brevis	Nil				Single unit only	
R pronator teres	Nil	N	N	N	N	N
R flexor pollicis longus	Nil	N	N	N	N	N
R tibialis anterior	Nil	N	N	N	N	N

↑, mildly increased; R, right; N, normal.

same electrode over the same distance, implying selective slowing of median motor conduction which most likely reflects compression at the carpal tunnel. Pathologically this degree of slowing implies demyelination in addition to the severe axon loss. The slight slowing of conduction in the forearm segment of the right median nerve (recording the second lumbrical) most likely reflects loss of the fastest large diameter axons which usually determine the measured conduction velocity. In addition, conduction velocity is reduced slightly with ageing, and diabetics commonly show mild slowing.

EMG confirms very severe denervation of the abductor pollicis brevis, although there appears to be at least one surviving axon given that there is a motor unit action potential under voluntary control. This denervation is expected given the severe weakness and wasting. Median innervation to muscles proximal to the wrist remains normal, including the pronator teres and flexor pollicis longus, which helps confirm the lesion lies distal to the branches innervating these muscles. EMG of the other muscles sampled, including the tibialis anterior, is within normal limits for the patient's age—there are usually a few more polyphasic units seen in elderly subjects, but the pattern of recruitment should remain essentially unchanged.

It is impossible to entirely rule out a mild axonal polyneuropathy in this patient since the normal range of sural and superficial peroneal sensory amplitudes decreases with age, but with considerable variation amongst normal volunteers. Over about 70 years of age the absence of lower limb sensory responses is not necessarily pathological, particularly if there is any ankle oedema. Likewise, in this age group a small CMAP from the extensor digitorum brevis is not a very robust marker of pathology since it may, for example, reflect trivial local nerve damage. In the case presented here it seems quite likely that he has a very mild sensory axonal neuropathy given his presentation. The finding of a reasonable amplitude ulnar sensory response (albeit slightly small), a normal CMAP from the extensor digitorum brevis, and normal EMG of tibialis anterior, all suggest that any generalized polyneuropathy must be mild.

Conclusion

There is neurophysiological evidence of an extremely severe median neuropathy at the right wrist, with very marked sensory and motor axon loss. In addition, although there is not convincing neurophysiological evidence, the findings are in keeping with the clinical suspicion of a mild length-dependent sensory axonal neuropathy.

Although his presentation is with a median neuropathy, given the severity of axon loss the expectations from treatment would need to be very guarded—it may well be possible to improve his pain, but muscle wasting and loss of sensation may well remain unchanged.

Comment: neurophysiological assessment of carpal tunnel syndrome

1. *The second lumbrical/interosseous study.* Because of their physical proximity, the CMAP from the median innervated second lumbrical and ulnar innervated interosseous muscles can be recorded from the same site in the palm (the interosseous response is probably a combination of the first palmar interosseous and the second dorsal interosseous muscle beneath it). Stimulation of the median then ulnar nerves at the wrist allows direct comparison of conduction in the two nerves provided there is an equal distance from either stimulation site to the active recording electrode (Fig. 14.2). This can be a valuable way of detecting slowing in the median nerve, which is most commonly at the carpal tunnel. A latency difference above 0.5ms is abnormal.

This method is particularly helpful in two situations. Firstly, in mild carpal tunnel syndrome it is a relatively sensitive test of mild slowing of median conduction. In this regard it provides similar information to other 'short segment

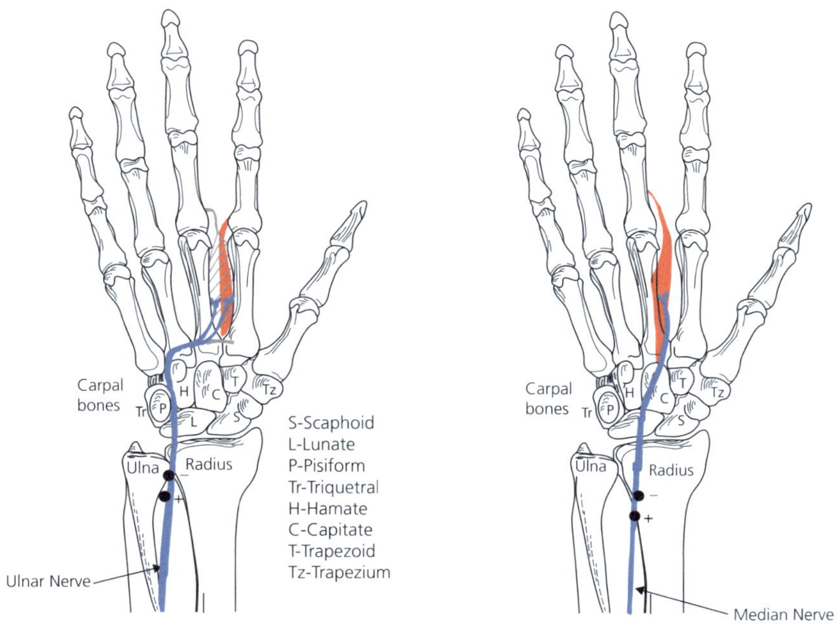

Figure 14.2 Lumbrical—interosseous conduction comparison.

studies', such as the comparison of latencies following median or ulnar nerve stimulation in the midpalm, recording at the wrist. Secondly, and probably more importantly, in very severe median neuropathies, such as the case presented here, median innervation to the second lumbrical is commonly preserved despite loss of the CMAP from abductor pollicis brevis, presumably because of fascicular damage to the median nerve. It therefore allows the detection of conduction slowing across the wrist, which helps localize the lesion.

2. *General principles: when the CMAP is very small or absent:*

a. Could it reflect a technical problem? If the patient can voluntarily move the muscle or there is a muscle twitch with stimulation there should be a CMAP recordable. Consider anomalous innervation if the equipment is working correctly but the muscle still cannot be stimulated.

b. Is there muscle wasting? Severe axonal injury results in wasting unless the process is acute. Distal conduction block or presynaptic neuromuscular junction failure can also result in a very small CMAP, but in these settings there is no wasting. Generally the CMAP is not very small even in severe myopathies or with postsynaptic neuromuscular junction disease.

c. What does the EMG show? Profuse fibrillations and positive sharp waves would support acute denervation, in which case there may be little wasting. If there are broad polyphasic motor unit action potentials the injury must be at least many weeks old given the time it takes for remodelling of the surviving motor units. A lack of spontaneous activity with reduced recruitment of relatively normal morphology motor unit action potentials is seen in motor conduction block, or very early axonal injury before fibrillations develop.

d. Is the finding clinically significant? For example, the extensor digitorum brevis and other intrinsic foot muscles can be denervated due to non-significant local trauma.

3. *Asymptomatic median neuropathies.* The finding of a mild asymptomatic median neuropathy at the wrist is common, especially in elderly or diabetic subjects, but may also be seen in association with amyloidosis, hypothyroidism, acromegaly, and a number of other predisposing conditions. It is frequently bilateral. If there are no associated symptoms the incidental finding should not be termed 'carpal tunnel syndrome' as this refers to a specific clinical presentation. The risk in not making this distinction is that surgery is erroneously undertaken.

4. *Assessing severity.* From a neurophysiological perspective there is generally a fairly orderly sequence of changes that occur as a focal entrapment

Table 14.11 Neurophysiological grading of the severity of focal entrapment neuropathy. Sensory and motor conduction measured across the lesion

	Sensory		Motor	
	Velocity	**Amplitude**	**Distal latency**	**Amplitude**
Very mild	Appropriate symptoms, no neurophysiological abnormality			
↓	↓	N	N	N
↓	↓↓↓	↓↓ or absent	↑ maybe	N
↓	Absent	Absent	↑↑↑	↓
Very severe	Sensory and motor responses both absent			

↓, mildly decreased; ↓↓, moderately decreased; ↓↓↓, severely decreased; ↑, mildly increased; ↑↑↑, severely increased; N, normal.

neuropathy increases in severity. To some extent this allows for grading of the severity of pathology, although occasionally lesions do not follow the expected sequence, depending on the aetiology and pattern of nerve damage (Table 14.11). Symptoms do not necessarily correlate with neurophysiological grade. However, such grading systems have some ability to predict the chance of successful symptom improvement following carpal tunnel release.

5. *Neurophysiology and surgery for carpal tunnel syndrome.* Although most cases of carpal tunnel syndrome are readily diagnosed clinically a substantial minority have an atypical presentation. This will of course impact on the effectiveness of treatment. Electrodiagnosis therefore has a role in establishing the diagnosis prior to surgery, and should be undertaken in all patients, particularly those with atypical symptoms or confounding pathology, or in whom the condition is thought to relate to occupational factors (there is some evidence for poorer treatment outcome in this group). Furthermore, electrodiagnostic grading of severity has a role in the assessment of patients prior to surgery since there is evidence that symptomatic improvement is less likely in very mild and very severe disease. It therefore allows a more informed discussion of the pros and cons of surgery. Most patients do not require postoperative nerve conduction studies since the degree of resolution of neurophysiological abnormalities is somewhat variable. For the small number of patients in whom surgery is not effective (up to 10–15%) repeat postoperative nerve conduction data is useful to help determine whether decompression is likely to have been adequate—nerve conduction parameters tend to improve, but not always back to normal, so lack of improvement suggests inadequate decompression. Management of these cases is extremely challenging without preoperative data.

Role of nerve conduction/EMG studies—suspected carpal tunnel syndrome

- All patients should have nerve conduction studies prior to surgery.
- Confirm the diagnosis by localizing the lesion and excluding mimicking disease, such as a C6 radiculopathy or other neuropathy (electroclinical diagnosis is better than clinical diagnosis alone).
- Assess severity, thereby helping to guide treatment choice and expectations from surgery (best symptomatic results from surgery are with moderate severity electrophysiological abnormality).
- Management of patients with residual symptoms after surgery: comparison of postoperative to preoperative nerve conduction parameters helps determine whether decompression was adequate.
- Patients who are not being treated surgically do not necessarily need nerve conduction studies unless their symptoms are atypical.

Limitations of nerve conduction/EMG studies—suspected carpal tunnel syndrome

- Incidental findings must not be over interpreted (over treated). Neurophysiological confirmation of a median neuropathy at the wrist must be accompanied by appropriate symptoms in order to be termed carpal tunnel syndrome.
- It is extremely difficult to interpret neurophysiological findings if they are first performed following an operation that has failed to relieve symptoms. Preoperative testing is recommended for all patients.
- Very mild pathology may cause significant symptoms yet pass undetected by nerve conduction studies. Normal results do not rule out carpal tunnel syndrome, but the diagnosis and treatment should be reconsidered.

Case 6

Clinical presentation

A 23-year-old gunner had been involved in a landmine blast in Iraq 2 months previously. At the time of the explosion he had been driving a small semi-armoured vehicle, and had sustained injury to the mid right thigh, probably from the impact of the door of the vehicle, as well as what appeared to be relatively minor shrapnel injury. There was no major vascular injury, but he underwent emergency stabilization of his fractured right femur. Following repatriation he underwent further surgery to the right femur, during which the sciatic nerve was visualized and appeared intact and without major injury or external compression.

He is now referred 2 months after the injury with a residual severe right foot drop. There is no convincing movement on attempted ankle dorsiflexion and eversion, but only relatively mild weakness of plantarflexion and inversion (both MRC grade 4). Knee flexion is limited by discomfort. There is numbness of the dorsum of the right foot, lateral lower leg and, to a lesser extent, the sole. The neurophysiological examination was requested to confirm the severity of injury and try to assist with prognosis and management. For results of nerve conduction studies and EMG see Tables 14.12 and 14.13.

Questions

1. Can you explain this pattern of injury?
2. Should EMG and nerve conduction studies be performed early after traumatic nerve injury?

Interpretation

Initial treatment was of course directed at stabilizing the patient, coping with vascular and bony injury. The subsequent pattern of weakness on clinical examination suggests severe damage to the peroneal nerve, with no proof from routine clinical examination that the nerve remains in continuity given the lack of ankle dorsiflexion and eversion. In addition there is weakness, albeit relatively mild, in the distribution of the tibial nerve. Clinical findings therefore suggest that the blast injury to the right thigh probably caused sciatic nerve damage, preferentially affecting the peroneal division.

EMG was requested to see whether there is proof that the peroneal nerve is in continuity, and therefore whether clinical improvement might be anticipated with conservative management. Furthermore, it was requested to determine the degree of tibial nerve injury since pain limited the clinical assessment, and

Table 14.12 Nerve conduction studies

Nerve	Stimulation	Recording	Amplitude (μV or mV)			Onset latency (ms)			Conduction velocity (m/s)			F wave latency (ms)		
			R	L	N	R	L	N	R	L	N	R	L	N
Sensory														
Sural	Calf	Posterior ankle	6	21	**≥10**			**≤3.8**	40	44	**≥40**			
Superficial peroneal	Lateral ankle	Dorsum of foot	Absent	14	**≥5**			**≤3.8**		43	**≥40**			
Motor														
Tibial	Ankle	AH	3.1	11.2	**≥4**	4.7	4.2	**≤5.8**						**≤56**
	Knee	AH	2.4	10.6					39	44	**≥41**			
Peroneal	Ankle	EDB	Absent	4.3	**≥2**		4.0	**≤6.5**		40				**≤56**
	Fibular head	EDB	Absent	4.0							**≥41**			
Peroneal	Fibular head	TA	Absent											

Sensory amplitudes are μV, motor amplitudes mV. R, right; L, left; N, normal; AH, abductor hallucis brevis; EDB extensor digitorum brevis; TA, tibialis anterior.

Table 14.13 EMG

Muscle	Spontaneous activity	Motor unit action potential			Recruitment	Interference pattern
		Duration	Amplitude	Phases		
R tibialis anterior	2+ fibs, PSW				Single motor unit active	
R peroneus longus	3+ fibs				No motor units activated	
R short head biceps femoris	2+ fibs				Single motor unit active	
R medial gastrocnemius	Nil	↑	↑	↑	Reduced	↓
R tibialis posterior	Nil	↑	N	↑	Reduced	↓
R vastus medialis	Nil	N	N	N	N	N
R gluteus medius	Nil	N	N	N	N	N

↑, mildly increased; ↓, mildly decreased; R, right; N, normal; fibs, fibrillation potentials; PSW, positive sharp waves.

since tibial innervated muscles might in due course be considered for tendon transfer if there was still no dorsiflexion in the months ahead.

The absence of the right superficial peroneal sensory response is consistent with severe axon loss. However, the right sural sensory response remains present, although small, proving that a proportion of sensory axons running via the tibial nerve remain in continuity with their cell bodies, through the level of the lesion in the thigh.

Motor responses confirm the same pattern of abnormality, with no CMAP recordable from the right extensor digitorum brevis or tibialis anterior muscles, both innervated by branches of the peroneal nerve. In contrast, a small CMAP was obtained from the abductor hallucis brevis, innervated via the tibial nerve.

EMG shows many fibrillation potentials and positive sharp waves in peroneal nerve territory, and a single motor unit action potential was found under voluntary control in the tibialis anterior. This must represent a surviving motor axon rather than one that has regenerated since it is too far from the level of injury to have reached this site at a growth rate of 1–2mm/day. Furthermore, it had the wrong morphology for a nascent motor unit action potential, being rather too high amplitude, broad, and polyphasic, suggesting many muscle fibres are innervated due to sprouting of additional terminal fibres from an existing motor neuron. Muscles innervated by the tibial division of the sciatic nerve show changes suggestive of mild partial denervation.

The fact that there are functioning motor axons in both tibial and peroneal branches of the sciatic nerve distal to the lesion proves both divisions of the nerve remain in continuity to some extent. Injury is likely to involve significant axonotmesis, suggesting there should be gradual recovery of at least some function with slow axon regeneration. In contrast, if there had been no EMG evidence of motor units under voluntary control, nerve continuity would not be proven. In this setting the neurophysiology cannot distinguish complete neurotmesis from axonotmesis, the concern being that the former would not recover without surgical repair. For completeness the electromyographer confirmed a normal EMG examination of the right gluteus medius, helping to exclude proximal plexus or root pathology—as expected clinically.

The pattern of sciatic nerve injury seen here is relatively common, with greater peroneal than tibial nerve involvement, although of course the mode of injury is unusual. This pattern of injury probably arises because the peroneal nerve lies superficially and is relatively tethered at the knee, so more susceptible to stretch in the thigh than the tibial nerve (for example, during difficult hip surgery). Its susceptibility may also result from differences in internal structure of the nerve, such as the course and orientation of axons plus their blood supply. The slight surprise in this case is that injury results from a bomb blast, which may not involve stretch, so the susceptibility of peroneal fibres may simply reflect their lateral position within the sciatic nerve, taking the full brunt of a compression injury and partly protecting the tibial fibres.

In light of the neurophysiological findings, and in this case also the surgical confirmation that there was no external compression of the affected sciatic nerve, the decision was taken to manage the patient conservatively. A repeat neurophysiological examination was performed 6 months later. In this study there was EMG evidence of regenerating axons beginning to reinnervate the short head of the biceps femoris, resulting in 'nascent' looking motor unit action potentials which are low amplitude, polyphasic, and often contain satellite potentials on EMG.

Conclusion

The neurophysiological examination confirms injury to the sciatic nerve in the thigh causing severe, but not complete, axon loss in the peroneal division, and moderate axon loss in the tibial division of that nerve. The peroneal nerve is proven to remain in continuity, so in the absence of external compression clinical recovery would be expected over several months, although the time course and eventual extent of recovery is not accurately predicted.

Comment: neurophysiological assessment of acute nerve injury

1. *Early, first few days to about 2–3 weeks.* EMG can sometimes help guide surgical decisions when there has been a severe injury resulting in complete absence of discernible muscle function, and when early surgical nerve repair is considered. In this instance, if EMG confirms that even one or two motor units remain under voluntary control distal to the lesion, it proves the nerve has not been completely transected, thus potentially avoiding nerve exploration depending on the clinical context.

A few days is not sufficient time for Wallerian degeneration in response to axon injury, thus early nerve conduction studies will be normal provided both stimulation and recording sites lie distal to the injury. Of course if the site of injury lies between the stimulating and recording electrodes the response will be small or absent even immediately after injury. At this early time point the reduction in response amplitude could in theory reflect conduction block or axon loss. It is too early for EMG to tell them apart since there would not have been sufficient time to develop fibrillation potentials, and any surviving motor unit action potentials would have normal morphology because it is far too early for there to have been motor unit remodelling.

2. *Subacute, three to several weeks.* During this period the neurophysiological examination can help determine the extent and type of nerve injury and its severity because there has been ample time for Wallerian degeneration. Thus sensory and motor response amplitudes will have decreased in proportion to the amount of axonal injury, and there will be fibrillation potentials on needle EMG of denervated muscle. Some indication of the expected time course of recovery can often be given, depending on the degree of conduction block (relatively rapid recovery) and axon loss (slower recovery) and the distance between site of injury and target muscle. Unfortunately nerve injury is often mixed, making prediction of rate and extent of recovery unreliable.

3. *Late, several weeks to many months after injury.* Usually late examinations are requested to assess if there is evidence of nerve regeneration when there is no discernible muscle contraction on clinical examination. Small polyphasic ('nascent') motor unit action potentials are seen as motor axons arrive and reinnervate the first few muscle fibres. Muscles close to the regenerating stump are reinnervated first. Signs of nerve regeneration include a Tinel's sign when tapping over the site of the advancing axon growth cones, and nascent units on EMG, provided the nerve contacts muscle fibres. If there is absolutely no evidence of nerve regeneration despite allowing adequate time at a rate of 1–2mm/day, there may be other surgical approaches to consider. These include operations directly on the nerve or compressing lesions, or tendon transfer from adequately innervated muscles (assessed by EMG if necessary) to try to re-establish essential movement or stabilize joints.

Role of nerve conduction/EMG studies in traumatic nerve injury

- Early (0–3 weeks): in muscles without discernible contraction voluntary EMG activity distal to the lesion confirms that the nerve remains in continuity, which may be sufficient to avoid acute surgical intervention.
- Subacute (3–6 weeks): the distribution, type and severity of nerve injury can be determined, and often a likely prognosis for recovery suggested.
- Late (months): EMG signs of nerve regeneration may be found in muscles with no apparent contraction, helping with management and planning late surgery.

Limitations of nerve conduction/EMG studies in traumatic nerve injury

- The distribution and severity of nerve injury cannot be accurately determined early (within 2–3 weeks) because of the time course of Wallerian degeneration.
- The presence of EMG activity under voluntary control distal to the lesion proves the nerve is in continuity. However, its absence does not prove that the nerve has been transected, or even that there is complete loss of axon integrity, since there may be conduction block.
- Prognosis for recovery depends on determining type, site and severity of nerve injury: conduction block is favourable, severe axon loss suggests a slow recovery, nerve root avulsion carries a poor prognosis, and so on. If pathology is mixed the prediction of rate and extent of recovery is inaccurate.
- Nerve conduction studies and EMG provide less information about sensory than motor nerve abnormality, and recovery, after traumatic nerve injury.

Case 7

Clinical presentation

A 16-year-old boy is referred with suspected Guillain–Barré syndrome. He gives an 8-day history of progressive weakness and sensory disturbance which initially affected his legs then progressed to involve his arms. He also complains of back pain. There was no preceding illness, and he is normally fit and a keen footballer. Examination reveals he is slightly underweight and has fairly symmetrical weakness, most severe distally (MRC grade 4 ankle plantar- and dorsiflexion, grade 4 finger abduction, and grade 4+ hip flexion). Deep tendon reflexes are absent. For results of nerve conduction studies and EMG see Tables 14.14 and 14.15.

Questions

1. Does the neurophysiology support the clinical suspicion of Guillain–Barré syndrome?
2. Is the pathology axonal or demyelinating?

Interpretation

Sensory responses from the upper limb, especially median and ulnar nerves, are slightly small, in contrast to the response from the sural nerves which are within normal limits. These findings suggest there is postganglionic upper limb pathology, either partial axon loss or possibly partial conduction block or temporal dispersion between the site of the stimulating and recording electrodes. It must be remembered that the study was performed only 8 days into the course of the illness. At this stage sensory axon loss may not be accurately reflected in the amplitude of sensory responses because of the time course of Wallerian degeneration. This pattern of relative preservation of sural sensory responses is quite common in Guillain–Barré syndrome, and unlike other length-dependent neuropathies.

Motor conduction shows slightly small CMAPs, with absent tibial and ulnar F-waves. However, there is only mild conduction slowing and mild prolongation of distal motor latencies. There was no significant temporal dispersion of motor responses, and no proven conduction block. Early in Guillain–Barré syndrome, particularly with mild disease, it is not uncommon to have relatively normal neurophysiology, or only mild changes such as loss of F-wave responses.

Considered in isolation, the slight reduction in CMAP amplitude could in theory be due to abnormality of the nerve, neuromuscular junction or, far less

Table 14.14 Nerve conduction studies

Nerve	Stimulation	Recording	Amplitude (μV or mV)			Onset latency (ms)			Conduction velocity (m/s)			F wave latency (ms)		
			R	L	N	R	L	N	R	L	N	R	L	N
Sensory														
Median	Middle finger	Wrist	5	4	**≥7**			**≤3.5**	50	46	**≥49**			
Ulnar	Little finger	Wrist	4	3	**≥5**			**≤3.1**	51	40	**≥49**			
Radial	Forearm	Snuff box	17		**≥12**			**≤3.0**	57		**≥50**			
Sural	Calf	Posterior ankle	19	18	**≥10**			**≤3.8**	45	43	**≥40**			
Superficial peroneal	Lateral ankle	Dorsum of foot	8		**≥5**			**≤3.8**	39		**≥40**			
Motor														
Median	Wrist	APB	4.5	5.4	**≥4**	4.3	3.9	**≤4.2**				30		**≤31**
	Elbow	APB	4.1	5.6					44	47	**≥49**			
Ulnar	Wrist	ADM	3.9		**≥6**	4.1		**≤3.3**				Absent		**≤32**
	Below elbow	ADM	3.4						43		**≥49**			
	Above elbow	ADM	3.3						45					
Tibial	Ankle	AH	4.5		**≥4**	6.5		**≤5.8**				Absent		**≤56**
	Knee	AH	3.4						33		**≥41**			

Sensory amplitudes are μV, motor amplitudes mV. R, right; L, left; N, normal; APB, abductor pollicis brevis; ADM, abductor digiti minimi; AH, abductor hallucis brevis.

Table 14.15 EMG

Muscle	Spontaneous activity	Motor unit action potential			Recruitment	Interference pattern
		Duration	Amplitude	Phases		
R 1st dorsal interosseous	Nil	N	N	N	Reduced	↓
R deltoid	Nil	N	N	N	Borderline	↓
R rectus femoris	Nil	N	↑	N	Mildly reduced	↓
R tibialis anterior	Nil	N	N	N	Reduced	↓↓

↑, mildly increased; ↓, mildly decreased; ↓↓, moderately decreased; R, right; N, normal.

likely, the muscle itself (excluding technical reasons for a small CMAP). In this context, however, with strong clinical suspicion of Guillain–Barré syndrome, the likely cause is either distal partial conduction block or axon loss. The mild prolongation of distal motor latencies is suggestive of distal nerve pathology, and in Guillain–Barré syndrome conduction block may occur beyond the most distal point of stimulation, where the blood–nerve barrier is weak. Since it is so distal, block at this site is not detected in the usual way on routine motor conduction studies. If the pathology is axonal it is still slightly too early to be confident that Wallerian degeneration, and the consequent reduction in CMAP amplitude, is complete. The absence of tibial and ulnar F-wave responses suggests that pathology also affects more proximal nerve segments, and favours dysfunction of the myelin rather than axonal degeneration, although of course the two pathologies can coexist.

EMG shows no spontaneous activity in the muscles examined, but, with the possible exception of very proximal muscles, fibrillation potentials are unlikely to be seen by day 8 even in the presence of motor axon degeneration, so their absence cannot be taken as evidence against axonal pathology. Recruitment of motor units is reduced, as is the interference pattern, consistent with either acute partial axon loss or conduction block reducing the available pool of motor units. These two are usually distinguished by the presence of spontaneous fibrillation potentials several days after axonal injury, followed eventually by motor unit remodelling, but at this early stage in the disease these changes would not be expected.

A follow up study a couple of weeks after initial presentation would provide further information about whether there is axon loss because fibrillation potentials would be expected. By this stage Wallerian degeneration would be complete, and therefore axon loss would be reflected by sensory and motor response amplitude reduction. Furthermore, over time nerve conduction changes suggestive of demyelination may become more apparent.

Conclusion

There is evidence of a non-length-dependent sensorimotor neuropathy which supports the clinical suspicion of Guillain–Barré syndrome. Despite the lack of severe conduction slowing or block there is some neurophysiological evidence to suggest demyelination is likely. Given the study was performed 8 days after symptom onset, the degree of axonal pathology cannot be determined.

Comment: the neurophysiology of Guillain–Barré syndrome

1. *Nerve susceptibility and the blood–nerve barrier.* In Guillain–Barré syndrome nerves tend to be affected early where the blood–nerve barrier is poor, both

proximally, at the nerve roots, and distally, near the neuromuscular junction. Proximal pathology is believed to contribute to early loss of f-waves, but it is possible for pathology at the nerve roots to remain completely undetected by routine nerve conduction studies, particularly since muscles and nerves are supplied by more than one root. In contrast, very distal motor conduction block will result in a loss of CMAP amplitude, as discussed later in this section. Characteristic findings suggestive of demyelination such as conduction slowing, prolongation of distal motor latency, temporal dispersion or more proximal conduction block may be absent, or apparent only after several days. In some cases the neurophysiology can be entirely normal when performed early in relatively mild disease.

2. *Conduction block versus axonal pathology.* Usually motor conduction block is detected by a loss of CMAP amplitude with proximal stimulation compared to distal stimulation below the site of block. However, with the very distal site of conduction block sometimes seen in Guillain–Barré syndrome there is no chance of stimulating distal to it, thus nerve conduction studies reveal a small amplitude CMAP which remains constant at all the usual sites of stimulation. This distal conduction block is hypothesized to relate to antibody-mediated dysfunction of the nodes of Ranvier, disrupting sodium channels and resulting in inability to transmit the action potential. Recovery can potentially be rapid since there is dysfunction of the myelin rather than structural change. One confounding factor is that distal axon degeneration is also described, and may appear similar neurophysiologically. Distal conduction block can sometimes be distinguished from axon loss because fibrillation potentials will not develop as a result of block alone, so their detection suggests there is at least some axon loss. EMG may need to be repeated to allow time for Wallerian degeneration. In the case presented here it is not possible to exclude axon loss since the examination is relatively early, before EMG changes are likely.

3. *Pathology is neither uniform, nor length dependent.* Although the pathology in Guillain–Barré syndrome is frequently widespread it is often not clinically or electrophysiologically uniform. The early loss of F-waves and relative sparing of the sural sensory response confirm that pathology is not length dependent. Sural sparing may reflect preferential involvement of relatively small-diameter myelinated axons in Guillain–Barré syndrome. When there is partial motor conduction block the early involvement of small-diameter axons can potentially mean that small motor units, usually activated first with gentle contraction, are not activated. Instead, large-diameter motor axons are activated early, each supplying large numbers of muscle fibres, resulting in needle EMG appearances that at first glance may appear to suggest denervation since there are large motor unit action potentials relatively early in recruitment. There are not, however,

spontaneous fibrillation potentials, and motor unit action potentials are not polyphasic.

4. *Normal values.* The issue of normal values deserves mention here since the patient is young, thin, and has no previous medical history of note. In this situation it is common to record relatively high-amplitude sensory and motor responses, although there is no guarantee of a patient's premorbid scores without previous testing. In the case presented here the patient's normal sural sensory response may be 40uV, but since it has never been measured a recording of 19uV falls within the normal range even though it may be about half what it should be. The comparable issue in motor studies is, to some extent, overcome by needle EMG, since mild axon loss resulting in even a slight reduction in CMAP amplitude will be sensitively detected.

Role of nerve conduction/EMG in suspected Guillain–Barré syndrome

- Confirm the diagnosis and rule out mimicking conditions, especially other causes of acute neuromuscular weakness on intensive care.
- Determine the type of Guillain–Barré syndrome by looking for axonal versus demyelinating pathology, and the degree of sensory versus motor involvement.
- The sum of CMAP amplitudes can help quantify disease severity and provide some indication of prognosis.

Limitations of nerve conduction/EMG in suspected Guillain–Barré syndrome

- In the first few days after symptom onset the neurophysiology may be entirely normal or there may only be subtle abnormalities—consider repeating it.
- It may be difficult or impossible to determine the relative contributions of demyelination versus axon loss, particularly in the first week or two before Wallerian degeneration is complete.
- Neurophysiological assessment cannot reliably predict which of the patients presenting acutely will continue to deteriorate and who will run a subacute versus more chronic course.

Case 8

Clinical presentation

A 21-year-old man presents with at least a 6-year history of distal lower limb weakness and slight clumsiness but minimal sensory disturbance. He has always been poor at sport. Recently his fingers have also become mildly weak. He was adopted and can provide no medical history of his genetic family. Examination reveals pes cavus and mild distal weakness of the lower limb (MRC grade 4 ankle dorsiflexion, 4+ plantarflexion) but almost normal distal upper limb power. There is very mild distal lower limb muscle wasting. Deep tendon reflexes are absent. For results of nerve conduction studies and EMG see Tables 14.16 and 14.17.

Questions

1. What type of neuropathy does the patient have?
2. Is there axon loss, and why is this important?

Interpretation

The sensory responses are all absent, consistent with postganglionic pathology affecting sensory nerves. This is commonly because of peripheral sensory axon loss (a severe neuropathy) or sensory cell body pathology (a sensory neuronopathy), particularly given all nerves are affected. However, it is worth remembering that a reduction in sensory response amplitude could also result from demyelination causing temporal dispersion or conduction block between the stimulating and recording sites.

There is very marked slowing of motor conduction of a similar magnitude in all three nerves tested, suggesting a homogeneous process between nerves. Within a single nerve the prolongation of the distal motor latency is roughly in proportion to the slowing of conduction measured more proximally, suggesting the degree of slowing is relatively uniform along the length of the nerve as well as between nerves. Waveform inspection showed no evidence of motor conduction block or significant temporal dispersion of the CMAP with proximal stimulation. These findings show there is a severe demyelinating process which is homogeneous both between nerves and within a single nerve.

The single lower limb CMAP recorded is slightly small, but upper limb responses are relatively well maintained, suggesting there is little axon loss, which fits with the relative lack of muscle wasting. Since muscle strength and bulk is relatively well preserved the neurophysiologist would not expect to find small CMAPs, and if they did, a technical problem or anomalous innervation should be suspected.

Table 14.16 Nerve conduction studies

Nerve	Stimulation	Recording	Amplitude (μV or mV)			Onset latency (ms)			Conduction velocity (m/s)			F wave latency (ms)		
			R	L	N	R	L	N	R	L	N	R	L	N
Sensory														
Median	Middle finger	Wrist	Absent		**≥7**			**≤3.5**			**≥49**			
Ulnar	Little finger	Wrist	Absent		**≥5**			**≤3.1**			**≥49**			
Radial	Forearm	Snuff box	Absent	Absent	**≥12**			**≤3.0**			**≥50**			
Sural	Calf	Posterior ankle	Absent		**≥10**			**≤3.8**			**≥40**			
Motor														
Median	Wrist	APB	5.4		**≥4**	9.2		**≤4.2**	21					**≤31**
	Elbow	APB	5.0								**≥49**			
Ulnar	Wrist	ADM	4.9		**≥6**	8.8		**≤3.3**	18					**≤32**
	Elbow	ADM	4.1								**≥49**			
Tibial	Ankle	AH	2.2		**≥4**	12.6		**≤5.8**	15					**≤56**
	Knee	AH	2.0								**≥41**			

Sensory amplitudes are μV, motor amplitudes mV. R, right; L, left; N, normal; APB, abductor pollicis brevis; ADM, abductor digiti minimi; AH, abductor hallucis brevis.

Table 14.17 EMG

Muscle	Spontaneous activity	Motor unit action potential			Recruitment	Interference pattern
		Duration	Amplitude	Phases		
R 1st dorsal interosseous	Nil	N	N	N	N	N
R tibialis anterior	Nil	↑	↑	N	Reduced	↓
R vastus medialis	Nil	N	N	N	N	N

↑, mildly increased; ↓, mildly decreased; R, right; N, normal.

EMG shows changes consistent with mild chronic partial denervation of the right tibialis anterior, the most distal muscle tested, but other muscles remain within normal limits. This suggests there has been a small amount of secondary axon loss, which is common in chronic demyelinating neuropathies.

Conclusion

There is a homogeneous demyelinating sensorimotor neuropathy with severe conduction slowing and mild secondary axon loss. These findings are suggestive of a genetic demyelinating neuropathy—type 1 Charcot–Marie–Tooth (CMT) disease.

Comment: neurophysiology of Charcot–Marie–Tooth disease

1. *Homogeneous neurophysiology.* Hereditary demyelinating neuropathies characteristically have very homogeneous nerve conduction findings. Firstly, different nerves tend to be affected to a similar degree, therefore the magnitude of slowing in the commonly measured segments of one nerve match those measured in other nerves. Secondly, the degree of slowing is fairly homogeneous along the length of a nerve, so the prolongation of the distal motor latency is in proportion to the amount of conduction slowing measured more proximally. If F-waves are recordable these too will be slowed to the extent predicted by routine conduction studies. Thirdly, there is generally little evidence of temporal dispersion, a sign of variation in the severity of demyelination between different axons, and usually no conduction block, a sign of focal pathology.

2. *Hereditary versus inflammatory demyelination.* Generally the progressive and relatively distinct clinical presentation of inflammatory demyelinating neuropathies means they are not confused with genetic neuropathies. The neurophysiology also tends to be distinct, and is usually patchy in chronic inflammatory demyelinating polyneuropathies (CIDP). The degree of slowing is often less than in type-1 CMT, commonly more like 30–45m/s, with different nerves affected to a variable degree. Furthermore, conduction block and temporal dispersion are common in CIDP, as are other signs of patchy pathology such as disproportionate prolongation of distal motor latencies relative to more proximal conduction velocities, or delay of F-wave responses out of proportion to conduction velocities. Occasionally the neurophysiology can give a clue to the underlying pathogenesis, for example, disproportionately prolonged distal motor latencies are suggestive of antibodies to myelin-associated glycoprotein when found in the context of an elderly patient presenting with sensory loss, weakness, tremor, and unsteadiness of gait.

The distinction of inflammatory from hereditary demyelinating neuropathies is complicated by the existence of a number of types of 'intermediate CMT', in which motor conduction velocities are commonly about 30–40m/s, and in which it is increasingly recognized that temporal dispersion or conduction block may be seen. It is worth considering genetic tests for these intermediate forms of CMT in patients whose neurophysiology is suggestive of inflammatory disease, but who fail to respond to treatment.

3. *Weakness in hereditary neuropathies*. Pure homogeneous conduction slowing does not cause weakness, which is why patients with demyelinating CMT disease may present relatively late and remain strong. Much of the eventual weakness and disability reflects progressive secondary axon loss. Weakness accompanied by muscle wasting suggests axon loss, and is more characteristic of patients with type 2 (axonal) than type 1 (demyelinating) CMT, although the milder primarily axonal forms may also present late.

4. *Is there secondary axon loss*? The degree of secondary axon loss plays an important role in determining the accrual of disability in hereditary demyelinating neuropathies, and it can be useful to estimate the proportion of axons that have been lost (although in routine clinical practice there is little point in following this over time). Detection of axon loss by EMG is sensitive, but this is generally a poor method of quantifying the loss. In contrast the amplitude of sensory and motor responses allows reasonable estimation of axon loss, but this becomes unreliable in the presence of conduction block or temporal dispersion (as mentioned earlier, both are uncommon in hereditary demyelinating neuropathies). Another confounding factor is reinnervation and ongoing remodelling of motor units, which tends to preserve CMAP amplitude and area, limiting sensitivity of the CMAP as a marker of axon loss. Special tests designed to estimate the number of motor units can help, but are beyond the scope of this book.

5. *Is there demyelination in addition to axon loss?* In the case presented here the degree of conduction slowing, with preserved CMAPs, provides clear evidence of demyelination. But in severe axonal neuropathies it can be difficult to decide whether there is an additional demyelinating component. The rule of thumb is that even with severe axon loss the conduction velocity should not fall below 75% of the lower limit of normal as a result of loss of large-diameter axons alone. For the median nerve in the forearm, 38m/s has been used as a lower limit, velocities below this implying there must be some additional demyelination even when there is severe axon loss. Whilst this concept is useful, it is important to remember that when there is only mild axon loss (and near-normal response amplitude) the finding of moderate slowing of median nerve motor conduction, say to 42m/s, provides evidence of demyelination.

In reality, a judgement has to be made whether the amount of axon loss, reflected by loss of amplitude of the CMAP, corresponds to the degree of conduction slowing. Other factors such as temperature, age, and height should also be borne in mind as they all affect conduction velocity.

Role of nerve conduction/EMG in the assessment of neuropathies

- Diagnosis and classification:
  - Motor versus sensory.
  - Demyelinating versus axonal.
  - Distribution: homogeneous, length dependent, patchy, proximal, etc.
  - Small-versus large-diameter fibre involvement.
- Severity of the neuropathy.
- Follow up to monitor disease progression and help determine treatment or prognosis.
- Exclude unexpected pathology which may complicate the clinical presentation such as a myopathy or radiculopathy.

Limitations of nerve conduction/EMG in the assessment of neuropathies

- Mild axonal neuropathies may not be detected given the wide range of normal values, particularly in the elderly or if there is peripheral oedema.
- Small-diameter fibre neuropathies will not be detected by routine nerve conduction studies. Suspect this when a patient reports burning pain with preserved reflexes.
- The patchy neurophysiology characteristic of inflammatory neuropathies may be indistinguishable from rare intermediate forms of Charcot–Marie–Tooth disease.
- The ability to detect change over time is only as good as the test–retest variability in nerve conduction parameters (minimized by having the same examiner).

Case 9

Clinical presentation

A 53-year-old woman presents with a 2-month history of diplopia with possible day-to-day variation in degree of image separation. There is no history of limb weakness or dysphagia, and no significant previous medical history. Examination reveals slightly reduced right eye abduction with right lateral gaze. There is mild ptosis but no convincing limb or eyelid fatiguability. Serum antibodies to the acetylcholine receptor were not detected. She has noticed no definite benefit having started pyridostigmine 2 weeks ago. For results of nerve conduction studies and EMG see Tables 14.18 and 14.19. See Table 14.20 for repetitive stimulation and Table 14.21 for voluntary single-fibre EMG.

Questions

1. Is myasthenia confirmed, and if so, is it localized or generalized?
2. Does it matter that the patient was taking pyridostigmine?

Interpretation

Routine nerve conduction studies and EMG are normal, thus excluding a significant neuropathic or myopathic process, although neither would provide a good explanation of the symptoms. However, these routine studies help to confirm that the abnormality of single-fibre EMG discovered later in the examination is due to disease at the neuromuscular junction—some degree of abnormality may also be seen in neurogenic and myopathic conditions.

Repetitive nerve stimulation is strictly within normal limits since the maximum decrement in amplitude is less than 10%. However, the finding of mild decrement in CMAP amplitudes recording the upper trapezius muscle is suggestive that there may be an abnormality, particularly since examination of the raw traces showed that the minimum CMAP was on the fourth of a train of ten stimuli delivered at 3Hz, with subtle increment thereafter; a pattern typically found in myasthenia. Furthermore, and also typical of myasthenia, the early decrement in CMAP during a 3Hz train of stimuli repairs after brief contraction, so is not seen immediately after 10s of forceful muscle contraction. In myasthenics, the exhaustion of reserves of acetylcholine late after prolonged contraction usually results in exacerbation of the CMAP decrement with a train of stimuli. This is not convincingly seen in this case.

Table 14.18 Nerve conduction studies

Nerve	Stimulation	Recording	Amplitude (μV or mV)			Onset latency (ms)			Conduction velocity (m/s)			F wave latency (ms)		
			R	**L**	**N**	**R**	**L**	**N**	**R**	**L**	**N**	**R**	**L**	**N**
Sensory														
Median	Index finger	Wrist	12		**≥7**			**≤3.5**	53		**≥49**			
Ulnar	Little finger	Wrist	6		**≥5**			**≤3.1**	54		**≥49**			
Sural	Calf	Posterior ankle	10		**≥10**			**≤3.8**	39		**≥40**			
Motor														
Median	Wrist	APB	7.8		**≥4**	3.5		**≤4.2**	56					**≤31**
	Elbow	APB	7.7								**≥49**			
Tibial	Ankle	AH	9.5		**≥4**	4.5		**≤5.8**	41					**≤56**
	Knee	AH	9.3								**≥41**			

Sensory amplitudes are μV, motor amplitudes mV. R, right; L, left; N, normal; APB, abductor pollicis brevis; AH, abductor hallucis brevis.

Table 14.19 EMG

Muscle	Spontaneous activity	Motor unit action potential			Recruitment	Interference pattern
		Duration	Amplitude	Phases		
R orbicularis oculi	Nil	N	N	N	N	N
R deltoid	Nil	N	N	N	N	N
R upper trapezius	Nil	N	N	N	N	N
R first dorsal interosseous	Nil	N	N	N	N	N
R vastus medialis	Nil	N	N	N	Poor activation	↓

↓, mildly decreased; R, right; N, normal.

Table 14.20 Repetitive stimulation . Percentage decrement is measured between the first and fourth stimulus in a train of ten

Muscle	Initial CMAP (mV)	Decrement in CMAP amplitude at 3Hz, %	Decrement immediately after 10s contraction, %	Decrement 2min after 1min of contraction, %
R abductor pollicis brevis	7.7	3	2	Not done
R trapezius	6.1	7	2	8
R nasalis	2.1	4	Not done	Not done

R, right.

Table 14.21 Voluntary single-fibre EMG

Muscle	Number of pairs examined	Number of pairs showing blocking	Number of pairs with increased jitter	Mean MCD (μs)
R extensor digitorum communis	21	0	1	31
R orbicularis oculi	14	2	7	64

MCD, mean consecutive difference; R, right.

Single-fibre EMG of the orbicularis oculi is abnormal, with significantly increased jitter in many recordings and occasional blocking of neuromuscular transmission noted. In contrast, single-fibre EMG examination of extensor digitorum communis remains within normal limits, suggesting that the abnormality of neuromuscular transmission is not widespread. The upper limit of normal is for two of 20 pairs to show increased jitter, provided the average of all the mean consecutive differences also lies within normal limits. Given the suspicious findings from repetitive stimulation of the upper trapezius it is arguable that a proximal upper limb muscle should have been tested with single-fibre EMG to look for abnormality beyond the eyes, but the examination is relatively time consuming.

Conclusion

There is evidence of a postsynaptic abnormality of neuromuscular transmission to support the clinical suspicion of ocular myasthenia. There is limited evidence to suggest that the disease may extend beyond the extraocular muscles to proximal limb muscles, but the neurophysiological abnormalities are not generalized.

Comment: neurophysiology and myasthenia gravis

1. *Neurophysiological abnormalities in mild myasthenia.* The first neurophysiological abnormality detected in very mild myasthenia is an isolated mild increase in jitter recorded on single-fibre EMG. With increasing disease severity there is progressive reduction in the safety factor by which the end-plate potential exceeds the threshold for muscle fibre action potential generation, so jitter increases and eventually intermittent failure of neuromuscular transmission occurs, termed blocking. Repetitive nerve stimulation studies only become abnormal once there is a reasonable amount of blocking of neuromuscular transmission, since the CMAP represents the sum of a large number of single muscle fibre potentials. Many of these muscle fibres have to fail to activate in order to result in a reduction in the CMAP with repetitive stimulation, and to be detected clinically as weakness. It is therefore not surprising that single-fibre EMG is a more sensitive way of detecting abnormalities of neuromuscular transmission than repetitive nerve stimulation.

2. *Which muscle to test for myasthenia?* Most patients with myasthenia have an abnormal single-fibre EMG examination provided appropriate muscles are tested. An abnormal amount of variation in the time it takes for neuromuscular transmission, recorded by single-fibre EMG as increased jitter, does not cause clinically detectable weakness, and does not result in abnormal results from repetitive nerve stimulation. Weakness in myasthenia results from blocking of neuromuscular transmission, so to maximize the chance of detecting an abnormality the EMG examination should include weak muscles. For suspected ocular myasthenia, single-fibre EMG examination of the orbicularis oculi has been shown to provide excellent sensitivity even though the recti may be clinically most affected, resulting in diplopia. In ocular disease it may also be helpful to examine limb muscles to determine whether there is more widespread subclinical disease (detected as increased jitter) since this may help clinical management, and may herald the onset of limb symptoms. If single-fibre EMG of a weak muscle is normal the weakness cannot be attributed to dysfunction of the neuromuscular junction. If there is no clinical weakness it is important that adequate numbers of neuromuscular junctions are studied with single-fibre EMG to maximize sensitivity—20 pairs with voluntary activation, but more with stimulated single-fibre EMG since the latter only tests a single neuromuscular junction at a time.

3. *Stopping cholinesterase inhibitors.* Often patients with suspected myasthenia will already have started treatment with a cholinesterase inhibitor prior to referral for single-fibre EMG studies. Usually it is still possible to detect abnormalities of neuromuscular transmission if there is true underlying disease, since increased jitter may be reduced but is generally not entirely normalized. In very mild cases it can help to stop the drug before examination, but in general this is not necessary. If there is anxiety that stopping the drug may trigger an acute deterioration in the patient's condition it implies that their disease is not mild, thus it is unlikely that a reduction in medication would be needed for detection of an abnormality.

4. *Single-fibre EMG abnormalities are not specific to myasthenia.* Other diseases of the neuromuscular junction cause abnormal jitter and blocking, for example, congenital myasthenic syndromes, Lambert–Eaton myasthenic syndrome or the administration of neuromuscular blocking agents (a trap for the unwary on the intensive care unit). Furthermore, diseases which are not primarily thought to affect neuromuscular transmission can result in abnormal jitter, including neuropathies and myopathies. This is particularly true when there is active remodelling of motor units, in which case abnormal jitter and blocking is thought to reflect immaturity of the new neuromuscular junctions and terminal nerve sprouts. In practical terms this means it is sensible to perform nerve conduction and EMG to see if jitter and blocking can be attributed to disease of the muscle or nerve.

5. *Decrement on repetitive stimulation is not specific to myasthenia gravis.* Repetitive stimulation is often abnormal in myasthenia gravis when a weak muscle is tested, but, like single-fibre EMG, it can be abnormal in other conditions, both those that primarily affect the neuromuscular junction as well as some neuropathic and myopathic diseases. These of course generally present with different symptoms, so tend not to cause confusion, and the amount of decrement is often small in these settings. It is important to pay particular attention to the progressive change in CMAP morphology in a train of stimuli. In myasthenia gravis the CMAPs elicited by a train of stimulations follow a typical pattern, with minimum amplitude at about the fourth stimulation which is then generally followed by a slight increment. Furthermore, in myasthenia there is typically repair of this decrement if repetitive stimulation is repeated immediately after a brief period of contraction.

Role of nerve conduction/EMG in disorders of the neuromuscular junction

- EMG helps exclude other diseases, for example, denervation in patients with a bulbar presentation, or myopathies with some ocular presentations.
- The most sensitive neurophysiological test of abnormal neuromuscular transmission is single-fibre EMG.
- Single-fibre EMG can sometimes detect subclinical disease in strong muscles, thus potentially may detect more generalized disease in a patient with ocular symptoms.
- The pattern of neurophysiological abnormality usually suggests whether disease is pre- or postsynaptic.
- There is some evidence that single-fibre EMG can be used to track disease progression, but it is not generally used in this context outside clinical trials.

Limitations of nerve conduction/EMG in disorders of the neuromuscular junction

- Abnormalities of single-fibre EMG and repetitive stimulation may occur as a result of denervation, drugs blocking neuromuscular transmission, or other diseases affecting neuromuscular transmission. Abnormality is therefore not specific to myasthenia.
- It is fairly common for repetitive nerve stimulation studies to be normal in mild myasthenia—single fibre EMG is more sensitive, but may still be normal.
- Single-fibre EMG requires patient cooperation. This may be impossible in young children or on the intensive care unit, but stimulated single-fibre EMG techniques help.

Case 10

Clinical presentation

A 68-year-old woman presents with proximal weakness of both upper and lower limbs and mild back discomfort. She reports feeling exhausted and has lost nearly 10kg in weight. She first noticed mild weakness around her shoulders about 3 months previously. At that time it was noted that her eosinophil sedimentation rate was elevated, and she was treated with oral steroids for suspected polymyalgia rheumatica but her symptoms continued to progress. Examination reveals symmetrical proximal weakness of shoulder abduction (MRC grade 4+), and hip flexion (grade 4). Reflexes are present with reinforcement. She has mild ankle oedema. She was admitted, and EMG requested as part of her work-up. For results of nerve conduction studies and EMG see Tables 14.22 and 14.23.

Questions

1. Is the weakness and pattern of EMG findings likely to be secondary to steroid treatment?
2. Does the presence of some large motor unit action potentials in the right deltoid suggest there is additional neuropathic pathology?

Interpretation

Sensory responses from the upper limb are within normal limits for age. Although there was no response recordable from the right sural nerve this is probably not significant in view of the ankle oedema. Furthermore, the normal range of sural response amplitudes decreases with age, such that, by 68 years of age, some asymptomatic normal subjects have very low-amplitude responses. Thus the neurophysiology does not provide evidence of a large fibre peripheral neuropathy—and indeed the patient had retained ankle jerks, albeit with reinforcement. Motor conduction studies are normal, and add little to the diagnostic formulation.

As might be expected from the history, EMG is the most helpful investigation. The finding of low-amplitude, polyphasic, short-duration motor unit action potentials which recruit rapidly with weak muscle contraction is consistent with the clinical suspicion of a myopathy. Clinically, and on EMG, proximal muscles are most affected, including the paraspinals. There are quite a lot of fibrillation potentials, which are common in some myopathies (including necrotizing myopathies), but uncommon in many other myopathies. In particular, given the history in this case, neither polymyalgia rheumatica nor

Table 14.22 Nerve conduction studies

Nerve	Stimulation	Recording	Amplitude (μV or mV)			Onset latency (ms)			Conduction velocity (m/s)			F wave latency (ms)		
			R	L	N	R	L	N	R	L	N	R	L	N
Sensory														
Median	Middle finger	Wrist	7		**≥7**			**≤3.5**	54		**≥49**			
Ulnar	Little finger	Wrist	6		**≥5**			**≤3.1**	52		**≥49**			
Radial	Forearm	Snuff box	14		**≥12**			**≤3.0**	59		**≥50**			
Sural	Calf	Posterior ankle	Oedema		**≥10**			**≤3.8**			**≥40**			
Motor														
Median	Wrist	APB	6.1		**≥4**	3.2		**≤4.2**				27		**≤31**
	Elbow	APB	5.8						54		**≥49**			
Tibial	Ankle	AH	4.9		**≥4**	4.7		**≤5.8**				54		**≤56**
	Knee	AH	4.0						42		**≥41**			

Sensory amplitudes are μV, motor amplitudes mV. R, right; L, left; N, normal; APB, abductor pollicis brevis; AH, abductor hallucis brevis.

Table 14.23 EMG

Muscle	Spontaneous activity	Motor unit action potential			Recruitment	Interference pattern
		Duration	Amplitude	Phases		
R deltoid	2+ fibs	↓ (also a few broad)	↓ (also a few high amplitude)	↑↑	Rapid	Full, low amplitude
R triceps	2+ fibs	↓	↓	↑	Slightly rapid	N
R 1st dorsal interosseous	Nil	N	N	N	N	N
R rectus femoris	1+ fibs	↓	N	↑	Rapid	Full, low amplitude
R vastus medialis	Nil	↓	N	↑	Slightly rapid	N
R tibialis anterior	Nil	N	N	N	N	N
R lower thoracic paraspinals	2+ fibs					

↑ mildly increased, ↑↑ moderately increased, ↓ mildly decreased, N normal, fibs fibrillation potentials

steroid-induced myopathies are associated with profuse spontaneous EMG activity. In fact the EMG generally remains fairly normal in these conditions, with no appreciable change in motor unit action potential morphology or recruitment pattern either. The EMG findings in this case are not specific for aetiology but support the admitting neurologist's suspicion of polymyositis.

Some large motor unit action potentials are seen, particularly in the right deltoid, but this is not uncommon in myopathies in which there is a degree of remodelling of motor units, and in general does not imply additional neuropathic disease. On EMG the rectus femoris appears rather more affected than the vastus medialis. This may represent a sampling effect since only a small proportion of the muscle is examined, despite needle insertions at different depths and in different directions. However, if assumed to be a real difference it may help guide muscle biopsy.

Usually it makes sense to test the weakest muscle with EMG, especially if the clinical presentation is relatively subtle, since this is where the greatest abnormality will be found, and thus the sensitivity of the test maximized. In this example the weakest muscle may have been iliopsoas given the degree of weakness of hip flexion. However, it was not sampled since clear EMG changes were recorded elsewhere, and because it would not be the muscle of choice for biopsy. A decision was therefore made that it would not add significantly to the findings.

Conclusion

The EMG is consistent with a proximal myopathy, with spontaneous fibrillation potentials seen at rest. Although not specific, these findings support the clinical suspicion of polymyositis, and argue against polymyalgia rheumatica or a steroid-induced myopathy.

Comment: EMG and myopathies

1. *Myopathies with fibrillation potentials.* Profuse fibrillation potentials and positive sharp waves are most often seen in neurogenic conditions, but it is important they are not considered specific to this since they may also be seen in myopathies, particularly acute necrotizing myopathies. In this setting they may arise because muscle fibres become divided, leaving a distal section which becomes denervated. Alternatively the pathological process may interrupt small intramuscular nerve branches, causing distal denervation of a small number of muscle fibres. Thus, although fibrillations and positive sharp waves arise from denervated muscle fibres, this end point may be the result of pathology that is primarily myopathic.

Myopathies commonly associated with fibrillation potentials

- Inflammatory: polymyositis, dermatomyositis, inclusion body myositis.
- Critical illness myopathy.
- Rhabdomyolysis after trauma, prolonged unconsciousness.
- Metabolic: acid maltase deficiency, debrancher enzyme deficiency.
- Congenital: myofibrillary, centronuclear, nemaline.
- Infective: HIV, viral myositis.
- Amyloid, sarcoid.
- Toxic: statins, cyclosporine, colchicine, acute alcohol.

2. *Other spontaneous EMG activity and myopathies.* Myotonia is a useful EMG finding that helps narrow the differential diagnosis of a myopathy. Disease associations may be grouped according to whether or not there is also clinically evident myotonia. Myotonic discharges are rarely reported in severe axonal disorders too. Complex repetitive discharges can bear some similarity to myotonic discharges (and indeed used to be termed 'pseudo-myotonia'), yet they simply signify a chronic myopathic or neurogenic condition.

Myopathies with myotonic discharges on EMG

- *With clinical myotonia*: myotonic dystrophy 1 and 2, myotonia congenita, paramyotonia congenita.
- *No clinical myotonia*: hyperkalaemic periodic paralysis, polymyositis, acid maltase deficiency, Schwartz–Jampel syndrome, toxic (colchicine, statin), amyloid.

3. *'Neurogenic' EMG findings in myopathies.* Motor unit action potentials with high amplitude and long duration arise because of remodelling of motor units within the muscle. They reflect motor units where the axon has sprouted extra distal nerve branches to reinnervate muscle fibres that have become denervated. As explained earlier, intramuscular denervation

and the drive for motor unit remodelling can occur in some myopathies, and does not imply an additional neuropathic condition. Some myopathic conditions, for example, inclusion body myositis, seem particularly prone to developing high-amplitude, broad (remodelled) motor unit action potentials intermixed with the expected low-amplitude, short-duration, polyphasic 'myopathic' motor unit action potentials. The shape of motor unit action potentials should therefore not be described as 'neurogenic' or 'myopathic', since it is the company that these potentials keep, in other words the broader EMG and clinical findings, that determine whether pathology is likely to be neurogenic or myopathic. The finding of a proportion of large motor unit action potentials in the context of a myopathy suggests that the pathological process must be relatively chronic—it takes many weeks to months for remodelling of motor units.

Myopathies commonly associated with large motor unit action potentials on EMG

- Inflammatory: polymyositis, dermatomyositis, inclusion body myositis, HIV-associated myopathy.
- Dystrophies: facioscapulohumeral muscular dystrophy, Emery–Dreifuss muscular dystrophy, oculopharyngeal muscular dystrophy, Duchenne and Decker muscular dystrophy.
- Metabolic myopathies: acid maltase deficiency, carnitine deficiency, debrancher deficiency.
- Congenital myopathies: centronuclear myopathy, nemaline rod myopathy.

4. *Myopathies in which the EMG remains normal.* Many myopathies are generally not associated with fibrillation potentials, for example, many metabolic and endocrine myopathies (in some there may be abnormalities of motor unit action potential morphology, recruitment, and interference patterns). Furthermore, some myopathies, for example, steroid myopathies and the muscle wasting seen in chronic disease, cause relatively selective type II muscle fibre pathology. This passes relatively undetected by routine needle EMG because type II muscle fibres tend to be activated late, during relatively forceful

contraction, at a time when many motor units are already firing. Finally, for the EMG to show myopathic features there must have been some functional or anatomical remodelling of motor units. Myopathic processes that primarily affect muscle fibre excitability, such as the periodic paralyses, would not necessarily result in observable changes on routine EMG, except possibly during an attack or if a chronic myopathy develops.

5. *EMG and muscle biopsy.* EMG is sometimes performed prior to muscle biopsy, to help guide selection of a suitably affected muscle. It is important that the biopsy avoids the sites sampled with the needle since this can lead to difficulty in interpreting the histology. In a disease with symmetrical clinical presentation it is common practice to restrict EMG to one side of the body, so that the other is clear for muscle biopsy. In general, the information gained by biopsy is maximized by choosing a muscle clearly affected by disease but not end stage, by which time characteristic pathology may be lost.

6. *Evolution of EMG changes in necrotizing myopathies.* Spontaneous fibrillation potentials will generally be seen in the active stages of an inflammatory necrotizing myopathy. Eventually this active phase subsides, with disappearance of the spontaneous activity but persistence of some large motor unit action potentials generated by intramuscular remodelling of motor units. The active phase may recur, however, with recycling of a similar sequence of events (see Chapter 8), and reappearance of fibrilation potentials.

Role of EMG in myopathies

- Help determine the distribution of muscles affected in a myopathy, and select a suitably affected muscle for biopsy.
- The presence and type of spontaneous EMG activity, plus the severity and distribution of myopathic findings, may provide clues to the likely aetiology.
- Exclude neurogenic causes of weakness, for example, neurogenic scapuloperoneal syndromes. Some caution must be taken since large motor unit action potentials can be seen in myopathies.
- In a patient with an inflammatory myopathy who is deteriorating on steroids, profuse fibrillations on EMG would favour an active inflammatory condition, rather than a steroid-induced myopathy.

Limitations of EMG in myopathies

- EMG is not always needed, or helpful, in the diagnosis of myopathies, particularly where there is a genetic test.
- Normal EMG findings may be due to sampling bias, where patchy pathology passes undetected. A normal EMG does not exclude a myopathy.
- Some types of muscle pathology pass undetected, for example, selective type II muscle fibre pathology in steroid induced myopathies.

Glossary

action potential The brief regenerative electric potential that propagates along a single axon or muscle fibre membrane. An all-or-none phenomenon; whenever the stimulus is at or above threshold, the action potential generated has a constant size and configuration.

active electrode Synonymous with exploring electrode. *See* recording electrode.

amplitude With reference to an action potential, the maximum voltage difference between two points, usually baseline-to-peak or peak-to-peak. By convention, the amplitude of potentials which have an initial negative deflection from the baseline, such as the compound muscle action potential and the antidromic sensory nerve action potential are measured from baseline to the most negative peak. In contrast, the amplitude of a compound sensory nerve action potential, motor unit potential, fibrillation potential, positive sharp wave, fasciculation potential, and most other action potentials is measured from the most positive peak to the most negative peak.

anode The positive terminal of an electric current source.

antidromic Propagation of a nerve impulse in the direction opposite to physiologic conduction. Contrast with orthodromic.

axonal degeneration Degeneration of the segment of a nerve distal to the cell body with preferential distal pathology.

axonotmesis Nerve injury characterized by axon and myelin sheath disruption with supporting connective tissue (endoneurium) preservation, resulting in axonal degeneration distal to the injury site. Compare neurapraxia, neurotmesis.

baseline 1) The potential recorded from a biologic system while the system is at rest. 2) A flat trace on the recording instrument; an equivalent term, isoelectric line, may be used.

blocking Term used in single-fibre electromyography to describe dropout of one or more components of the potential during sequential firings. A sign of abnormal neuromuscular transmission, which may be due to primary neuromuscular transmission disorders, such as myasthenia gravis and other myasthenic syndromes. Also seen as a result of degeneration and reinnervation in neuropathies or myopathies.

cathode The negative terminal of an electric current source.

complex repetitive discharge A type of spontaneous activity. Consists of a regularly repeating series of complex polyphasic or serrated potentials that begin abruptly after needle electrode movement or spontaneously. May be seen in both myopathic and neurogenic disorders, usually chronic.

compound muscle action potential (CMAP) The summation of nearly synchronous muscle fibre action potentials recorded from a muscle, commonly produced by stimulation of the nerve supplying the muscle.

compound sensory nerve action potential (compound SNAP) A compound nerve action potential recorded from the afferent fibres of a sensory nerve, a sensory branch of a mixed nerve or in response to stimulation of a sensory nerve or a dorsal nerve root. Also referred to by the less preferred terms sensory response, sensory potential, or SNAP.

concentric needle electrode Recording electrode that measures an electric potential difference between a centrally insulated wire and the cannula of the needle through which it runs.

conduction block Failure of an action potential to propagate past a particular point in the nervous system whereas conduction is possible below the point of the block.

conduction distance The length of nerve or muscle over which conduction is determined, customarily measured in centimetres or millimetres.

conduction velocity (CV) Speed of propagation of an action potential along a nerve or muscle fibre. For a nerve trunk, the maximum conduction velocity is calculated in meters per second (m/s).

constructive interference The summation of two or more waveforms that are in phase, resulting in a compound waveform of higher amplitude than the individual waveforms.

decrementing response A reproducible decline in the amplitude and/or area of the M wave (the CMAP) of successive responses to repetitive nerve stimulation. A decrementing response with repetitive nerve stimulation commonly occurs in disorders of neuromuscular transmission, but can also be seen in some neuropathies, myopathies, and motor neuron disease.

demyelination Disease process affecting the myelin sheath of central or peripheral nerve fibres, manifested by conduction velocity slowing, conduction block, or both.

depolarization A change in the existing membrane potential to a less negative value. Depolarizing an excitable cell from its resting level to threshold typically generates an action potential.

destructive interference The summation of two or more waveforms that are not in phase, resulting in a compound waveform of lower amplitude than the individual waveforms.

distal latency The interval between the delivery of a stimulus to the most distal point of stimulation on a nerve and the onset of a response. A measure of the conduction properties of the distal most portion of motor or sensory nerves.

early recruitment A recruitment pattern which occurs in association with a reduction in the number of muscle fibres per motor unit or when the force generated by the fibres is reduced. At low levels of muscle contraction more motor unit action potentials are recorded than expected, and a full interference pattern may be recorded at relatively low levels of muscle contraction. Most often encountered in myopathy.

earth electrode Synonymous with ground electrode.

electromyography (EMG) Strictly defined, the recording and study of insertion, spontaneous, and voluntary activity of muscle with a recording electrode (either a needle electrode for invasive EMG or a surface electrode for kinesiologic studies).

end-plate activity Spontaneous electric activity recorded with a needle electrode close to muscle end plates.

end-plate noise A type of end-plate activity (monophasic).

end-plate potential (EPP) The graded non-propagated membrane potential induced in the postsynaptic membrane of a muscle fibre by release of acetylcholine from the presynaptic axon terminal in response to an action potential.

end-plate zone The region in a muscle where neuromuscular junctions are concentrated.

F-wave An action potential evoked intermittently from a muscle by a supramaximal electric stimulus to the nerve due to antidromic activation of motor neurons.

fasciculation The random, spontaneous twitching of a group of muscle fibres belonging to a single motor unit. The twitch may produce movement of the overlying skin. The electric activity associated with the twitch is strictly termed a fasciculation potential, but often referred to as a fasciculation.

fasciculation potential The electric activity associated with a fasciculation which has the configuration of a motor unit activation potential but which occurs spontaneously.

fibrillation The spontaneous contractions of individual muscle fibres which are not visible through the skin. This term has been used loosely in electromyography for the preferred term, fibrillation potential.

fibrillation potential The action potential of a single muscle fibre occurring spontaneously or after movement of a needle electrode. Usually fires at a constant rate.

frequency Number of complete cycles of a repetitive waveform in 1 second. Measured in hertz (Hz) or cycles per second (cps or c/s).

ground electrode A connection from the patient to earth. Used as a common return for an electric circuit and as an arbitrary zero potential reference point.

H-wave A compound muscle action potential with a consistent latency recorded from muscles after stimulation of the nerve. Regularly found in adults only in a limited group of physiologic extensors, particularly the calf muscles. Most reliably elicited with a stimulus of long duration (500–1000μs). A stimulus intensity sufficient to elicit a maximal amplitude M-wave reduces or abolishes the H-wave.

hyperpolarization A change in the existing membrane potential to a more negative value.

inching A nerve conduction study technique consisting of applying stimuli at multiple short distance increments along the course of a nerve. This technique is used to localize an area of focal slowing or conduction block.

incrementing response A reproducible increase in amplitude and/or area of successive M waves to repetitive nerve stimulation.

insertion activity Electric activity caused by insertion or movement of a needle electrode within a muscle.

interference pattern Electric activity recorded from a muscle with a needle electrode during maximal voluntary effort. A full interference pattern implies that no individual motor unit action potentials can be clearly identified.

jiggle Shape variability of motor unit action potentials recorded with a conventional EMG needle electrode. A small amount occurs normally. In conditions of disturbed neuromuscular transmission, including early reinnervation and myasthenic disorders, the variability can be sufficiently large to be easily detectable by eye.

jitter The variability of consecutive discharges of the interpotential interval between two muscle fibre action potentials belonging to the same motor unit. Usually expressed quantitatively as the mean value of the difference between the interpotential intervals of successive discharges (the mean consecutive difference).

latency Interval between a stimulus and a response. The peak latency is the interval between the onset of a stimulus and a specified peak of the evoked potential.

M-wave A compound muscle action potential evoked from a muscle by an electric stimulus to its motor nerve. By convention, the M-wave elicited by a supramaximal stimulus is used for motor nerve conduction studies. Also referred to as the motor response.

mean consecutive difference *See* jitter.

miniature end-plate potential The postsynaptic muscle fibre potentials produced through the spontaneous release of individual acetylcholine quanta from the presynaptic axon terminal.

mixed nerve A nerve composed of both motor and sensory axons.

mononeuropathy Pathology affecting a single nerve.

motor latency Interval between the onset of a stimulus and the onset of the resultant compound muscle action potential (M-wave). The term may be qualified, as proximal motor latency or distal motor latency, depending on the relative position of the stimulus.

motor nerve A nerve containing axons which innervate extrafusal and intrafusal muscle fibres. These nerves also contain sensory afferent fibres from muscle and other deep structures.

motor response 1) The compound muscle action potential (M-wave) recorded over a muscle in response to stimulation of the nerve to the muscle. 2) The muscle twitch or contraction elicited by stimulation of the nerve to a muscle. 3) The muscle twitch elicited by the muscle stretch reflex.

motor unit The anatomic element consisting of an anterior horn cell, its axon, the neuromuscular junctions, and all of the muscle fibres innervated by the axon.

motor unit action potential (MUAP) The compound action potential of a single motor unit whose muscle fibres lie within the recording range of an electrode. Synonym: motor unit potential.

motor unit territory The area of a muscle cross-section within which the muscle fibres belonging to an individual motor unit are distributed.

muscle fibre action potential Action potential recorded from a single muscle fibre.

myokymia Continuous quivering or undulating movement of surface and overlying skin and mucous membrane associated with spontaneous, repetitive discharge of motor unit action potentials.

myokymic discharge A form of involuntary activity in which motor unit action potentials fire repetitively and may be associated with clinical myokymia.

myopathy Disorder affecting the structure and/or function of muscle fibres. Not all of these disorders show abnormalities on needle electromyography.

myotonia Delayed relaxation of a muscle after voluntary contraction or percussion. Associated with propagated electric activity, such as myotonic discharges, complex repetitive discharges, or neuromyotonic discharges.

myotonic discharge Repetitive discharge which wax and wane at rates of 20–80Hz following needle electrode insertion, voluntary muscle contraction, or after muscle percussion. Due to independent, repetitive discharges of single muscle fibres.

nascent motor unit potential Refers to very low-amplitude, short-duration, highly polyphasic motor unit action potentials observed during early states of reinnervation. Commonly used but this terminology is discouraged, as it incorrectly implies diagnostic significance of a motor unit action potential configuration.

nerve conduction velocity The speed of action potential propagation along a nerve fibre or nerve trunk. Generally assumed to refer to the maximum speed of propagation unless otherwise specified.

nerve fibre action potential Action potential recorded from a single axon.

neurapraxia Clinical term used to describe the reversible deficits produced by focal lesions of large myelinated nerve fibres due to conduction block. The axon and endoneurium are not injured at the lesion site.

neuromyotonia Clinical syndrome of continuous muscle fibre activity manifested as continuous muscle rippling and stiffness.

neuromyotonic discharge Bursts of motor unit action potentials that fire at high rates (150–300Hz) for a few seconds, often starting or stopping abruptly.

neurotmesis Partial or complete nerve severance including the axons and endoneurium, resulting in axonal degeneration distal to the injury site.

order of activation The sequence of appearance of different motor unit action potentials with increasing strength of voluntary contraction.

orthodromic Propagation of a nerve impulse in the same direction as physiologic conduction. Contrast with antidromic.

phase The fraction of a complete cycle that has elapsed as measured from a specified reference point. Generally measured in degrees.

plexopathy Pathology at the level of the plexus.

polyphasic action potential An action potential with four or more baseline crossings, producing five or more phases.

positive sharp wave A biphasic, brief positive then longer negative action potential of a single muscle fibre. It is initiated by needle electrode movement or occurs spontaneously.

postganglionic Pathology affecting nerves distal to the dorsal root ganglion.

preganglionic Pathology that affects nerves proximal to the dorsal root ganglion.

radiculopathy Pathology of the nerve roots.

recording electrode Device used to record electric potential difference. All electric recordings require two electrodes. The electrode close to the source of the activity to be recorded is called the active or exploring electrode (E-1), and the other recording electrode is called the reference electrode (E-2). By present convention, a potential difference that is negative at the active electrode relative to the reference electrode causes an upward deflection on the display screen.

recruitment The successive activation of the same and additional motor units with increasing strength of voluntary muscle contraction.

recruitment frequency Firing rate of a motor unit action potential (MUAP) when a different MUAP first appears during gradually increasing voluntary muscle contraction.

recruitment pattern A qualitative and/or quantitative description of the sequence of appearance of motor unit action potentials during increasing voluntary muscle contraction. The recruitment frequency and recruitment interval are two quantitative measures commonly used.

reduced recruitment pattern A descriptive term for the interference pattern when the number of motor units available to generate a muscle contraction are reduced.

repetitive nerve stimulation The technique of repeated supramaximal stimulation of a nerve while recording successive M-waves from a muscle innervated by the nerve.

resting membrane potential Voltage across the membrane of an excitable cell in the absence of a stimulus.

satellite potential A small action potential which fires in a time-locked relationship to the main action potential, separated from the main motor unit action potential by an isoelectric interval.

sensory potential Synonym for the more precise term, compound sensory nerve action potential.

single-fibre electromyography (sfEMG) The recording of single muscle fibre action potentials using a needle electrode. Permits accurate measurement of the timing of activation, and thus assessment of neuromuscular transmission.

small fibre Narrow-diameter nerve fibres that are thinly myelinated or unmyelinated. There are a number of types, and they carry pain and temperature information as well as autonomic functions.

spontaneous activity Electric activity recorded from muscle at rest after insertion activity has subsided and when there is not voluntary contraction or an external stimulus.

stimulating electrode Device used to deliver electric current. All electric stimulation requires two electrodes; the negative terminal is termed the cathode, and the positive terminal is the anode.

stimulation single-fibre electromyography Use of electrical stimulation instead of voluntary activation of motor units for the analysis of single-fibre electromyography.

temporal dispersion Relative desynchronization of components of a compound potential due to different rates of conduction of each synchronously evoked component from the stimulation point to the recording electrode.

threshold The level at which a clear and abrupt transition occurs from one state to another. The term is generally used to refer to the voltage level at which an action potential is initiated in an axon or muscle fibre.

voluntary activity In electromyography, the electric activity recorded from a muscle with consciously controlled contraction.

Wallerian degeneration Degeneration of the segment of an axon distal to nerve injury that destroys its continuity.

Modified from AAEM glossary of terms in electrodiagnostic medicine. *Muscle Nerve* 2001, **24** (Supplement 10), s5–s28.

Index

Note: Page numbers in **bold** are glossary entries

T

U

Made in the USA
Monee, IL
13 September 2026

62977357R00160